204

"This is a poignant and beautiful book about Japanese culture and spirituality. As prayer leads into play and vice versa, the book connects the lighthearted and delightful aspects of Japanese culture to the more serious and deeply felt elements of Japanese spiritual belief. I look forward to sharing this beautiful book with friends and colleagues."

—Susan Napier, author of *Miyazakiworld*

"Transcendently intimate . . . A personal journey of remembrance and healing leads to a heightened exploration of the mystic realms of Japan. Yoda provides insights into Japanese spiritual lore as well as practical lessons in opening yourself to comforting unseen presences that can change your life."

—Alfred Birnbaum, translator of Haruki Murakami's works and editor of *Monkey Brain Sushi*

"This intimate, often moving reflection on Japanese folkways promises a welcome guide to organizing messy feelings and finding joy in the larger world around us. Given the ongoing global upheaval, I was excited reading about her experiments in healing and self-care, through traditions we might otherwise never hear about."

—Charo B. D'Etcheverry, author of *Love After* The Tale of Genji

"Through her own spiritual development, Yoda skillfully unbundles the philosophical and habitual foundations of Japanese people. Most Japanese don't consider themselves religious, and yet their way of life manifests Shinto and Buddhist belief systems."

—Dr. Shizuka Modica, lecturer, UVA Darden School of Business

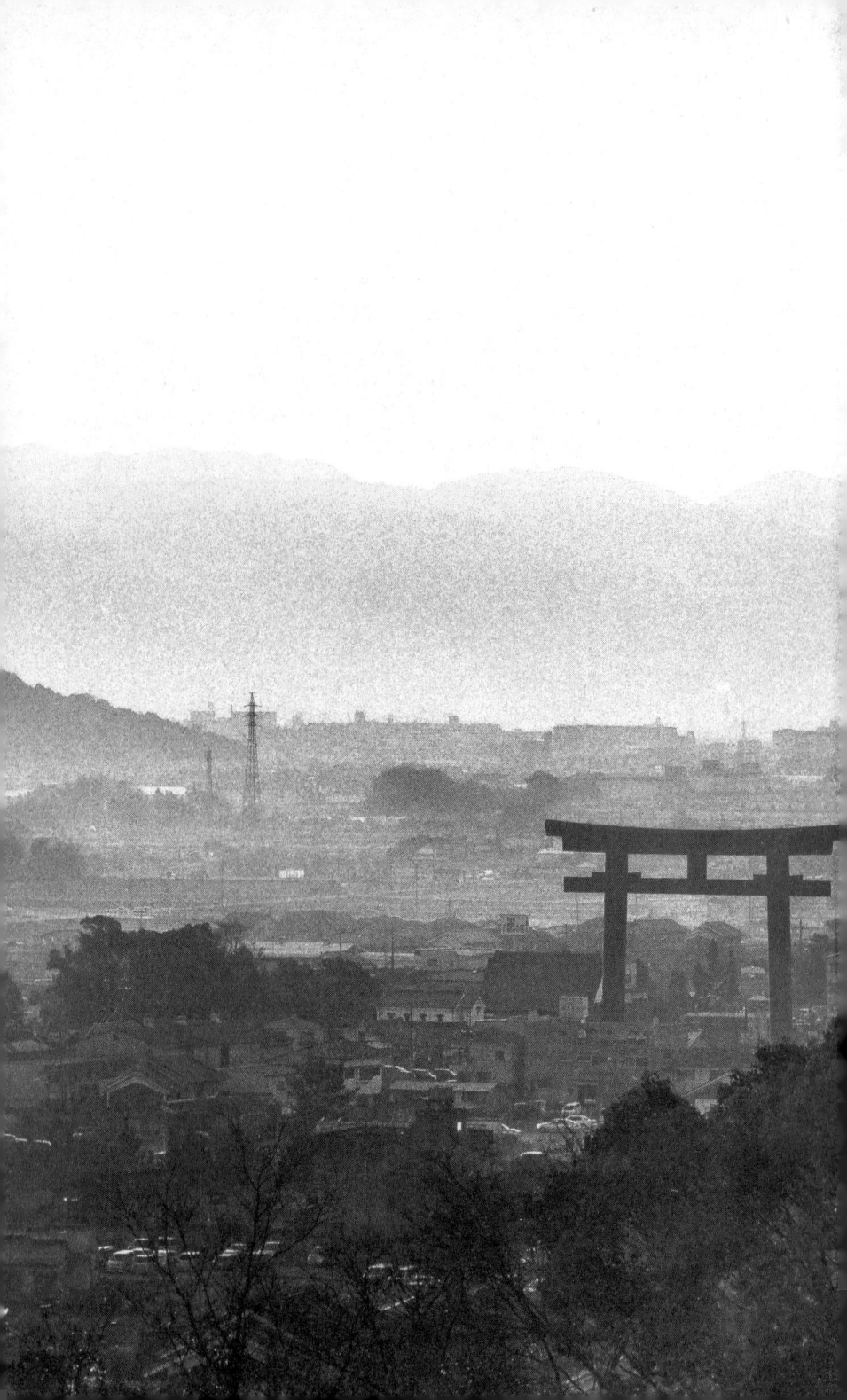

EIGHT MILLION WAYS TO HAPPINESS

Wisdom for Inspiration and Healing from the Heart of Japan

HIROKO YODA

Tiny Reparations Books

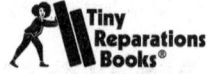

Tiny
Reparations
Books®

An imprint of Penguin Random House LLC
1745 Broadway, New York, NY 10019
penguinrandomhouse.com

Tiny Reparations and Tiny Reparations Books with colophon are
registered trademarks of YQY, Inc.

Book design by Shannon Nicole Plunkett

LIBRARY OF CONGRESS CATALOGING-IN-PUBLICATION DATA
has been applied for.

ISBN 9780593474433 (hardcover)
ISBN 9780593474440 (ebook)

Printed in the United States of America
1st Printing

The authorized representative in the EU for product safety and
compliance is Penguin Random House Ireland, Morrison Chambers,
32 Nassau Street, Dublin D02 YH68, Ireland, https://eu-contact.penguin.ie.

CONTENTS

Prologue • 1

Part One:
AWAKENING:
EIGHT MILLION KAMI • 25

CHAPTER 1:
The Invisibles: Shinto • 27

CHAPTER 2:
The Harmony of Conflict: Buddhism • 55

CHAPTER 3:
Making Friends with Monsters: Shugendo • 87

Part Two:
DARKNESS:
WALKING THROUGH HARDSHIP • 125

CHAPTER 4:
Angry Ghosts: Onryo • 127

CHAPTER 5:
Belief without Belief: Hanshin-Hangi • 154

CHAPTER 6:
Curating Your Rituals: Funeral Buddhism • 184

Part Three:
REBIRTH:
EVERYDAY SPIRITUALITY • 213

CHAPTER 7:
Love Will Travel: Kuyo • 215

CHAPTER 8:
Radically Inclusive: Kumano • 240

CHAPTER 9:
Prayer and Play: Asobi • 279

Epilogue • 329
Acknowledgments • 345
Notes • 347

EIGHT MILLION WAYS
TO HAPPINESS

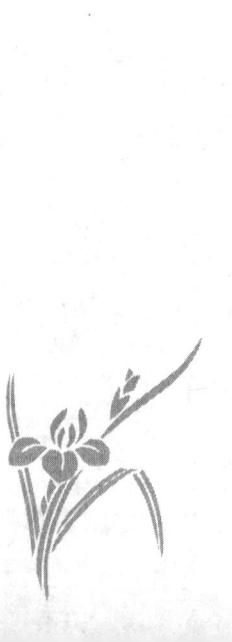

Prologue

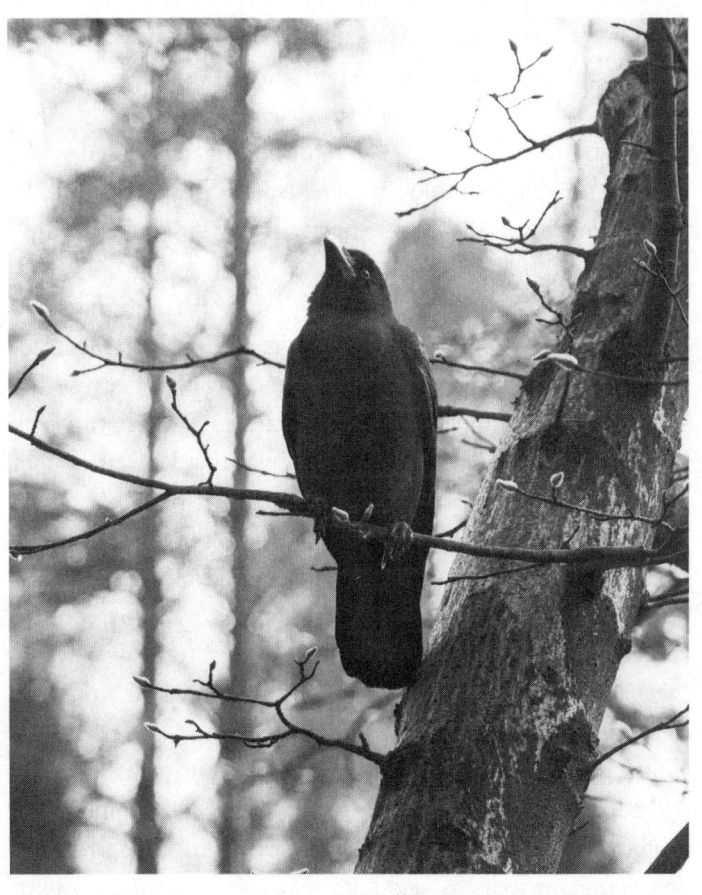

As the leaves began to fall from the trees one autumn, I found my own spirits sinking in turn. It was 2008, and it was supposed to be a celebratory time. My husband and I had just finished a book, a richly illustrated guide to creatures from Japanese folklore that took us years to create. But a few months after it was published, my mother passed away. I placed the very first copy we'd received from the publisher in her coffin. She had been so happy when she first saw it, even though she couldn't read English. She even told me that she was proud. When she was cremated, it went along with her to the land of the dead.

Shortly thereafter a close childhood friend passed without warning. Then Luke, our beloved family dog, died. In the space of a few months my string of farewells became almost too much to bear.

In my head, of course, I knew that everything that lives is destined to die. But that was, or had been, pure abstraction. I never thought about my parents' deaths, because the subject was unthinkable. Call it denial, call it what you will: It was so painful to contemplate seriously that I never thought seriously about it.

"If you want to do something nice for someone, you have to do it while they're still here," my mother once said to me during some long-ago argument. "It doesn't do any good to spread a comforter on a grave." We tussled so regularly that I can't even recall what we were fighting about, but the memory bubbled up from the depths after her passing. I think she was trying to tell me, in her own way, that we only had a limited amount of time together and so I should make the best of it. I knew she had lost her own mother when she was young, and she missed her greatly. But I wasn't ready to hear that then, and quickly shrugged it off, or rather, buried it deep within. Through thick and thin, anger and happiness, health and sickness, she and my father were just *there*, like the firmament above or the ground below, and I couldn't imagine otherwise. And if it (always *it*, my refusal to name the thing a kind of taming) did eventually happen, well, that would be a long way in the future. Until it wasn't.

My mother was an old woman who had been sick for many years, but even still, her death roiled me like nothing I had experienced. Day to day, I felt as though the flames of my soul had been snuffed, as though the world had drained of color. I began to question my own identity. I realized for the first time how much I had defined myself through my relationship to my mother. Sometimes, I felt that I knew myself through my dutifulness and affection toward her. Other times, perhaps more often than I liked, I seethed under a pall of injustice, anger, and opposition. But I always saw myself as part of a bigger system, a satellite in thrall to a star with an inescapable pull. Now that star was gone. In its place was a void with an even stronger, more dangerous gravity.

The subsequent deaths of my old friend and my dog only added to the disorientation. Loss became the lens through which I saw the world. I knew I would have to find a new way to define myself, but I had no idea how. I grew exquisitely sensitive. Words of comfort from well-meaning friends brought only pain; nobody could fill the new holes in my heart. Somehow, I sensed that only I could bring myself back together.

At some point I decided to take a long walk in the park. I had recently grown interested in photography, and carried my camera, a heavy digital single-lens reflex model that I'd purchased in hopes of refining my techniques. Sunk in my sorrow, however, I had no energy to see things through the lens. My walk was brief. I went out, head down, shuffled my feet, came home, and cried.

The cycle repeated over days and weeks. Gradually, I decided to make my walks a little longer. Then I resolved to keep my face up, looking ahead instead of looking down. Or I tried to, anyway. One day, I don't know how many later, I managed to do it. I looked up. And I saw something amazing.

A young raven rested on a branch, looking up to the sky. Its eyes looked sad to me, yet it kept its beak up, mesmerized as though looking at something magnificent. And it was: the sky, as large and free as it had ever appeared to me. It felt like the world stopped turning for a moment. Instinctively, I raised the camera and clicked the shutter. The frame was perfect, to me at least: sweet, bitter, sorrowful, beautiful, all at once.

The raven perched above a small but very old shrine. It was Shinto, with a series of tori'i gates standing astride the path leading inside. Once painted a fiery scarlet, the gates had faded to a dull vermilion from years of exposure to wind and rain. A series of stone slabs, their centers worn smooth from countless steps, led to the place of worship: a small roofed structure, just large enough for one person to enter, open to the elements, its pillars the same auburn hue as the gates.

Much later, I learned from old maps that the little shrine had been standing on this spot for more than 350 years. It must have been rebuilt over the centuries, as is custom, but not recently, judging from the condition of the stone, paint, and wood. This was a tiny, humble local spot for prayer, like countless others found throughout Japan. I'd passed by so many times before. Yet this time, I found myself transfixed. Boughs of Japanese maple swayed overhead, delicate leaves backlit by the autumn sun, dappling the stepping stones below with dancing sunlight. A soft breeze rose at my back, as though ushering me inside.

I raised my camera and took a shot. As a photographer, or more accurately someone who harbored aspirations of being one, I knew that this beautiful moment was an artifact of light. Light is the soul of photography; it is what imbues a two-dimensional image with drama and life. Outdoors, photographers are at the mercy of the sun, of the earth as it rotates on its axis, transforming the angle of light, degree by tiny degree throughout the seasons, never to repeat twice in precisely the same way.

On a moment-to-moment basis the shifts in the light are almost imperceptible. But the more time you spend behind a camera's viewfinder, the more you realize just how quickly the seemingly solid ground beneath our feet is moving. We are spinning through the cosmos on a journey plotted out long before any of us were born, or humans even walked the earth. So when I clicked my shutter in front of the tori'i gates, I was struck by the beauty of it all: not only the image, but the whole of it, the timing, the subject, the framing, the composition, the lighting. A combination of countless variables, a few under my control, a great many more not. The time of day and season, the wind's caress of the leaves, the subtle wear on the pillars and the checkerboard of light playing across them. Everything aligned for a split second. Then it was gone. As a photographer, I felt lucky to have captured a great shot. But deep inside I realized how much more was at play. That moment wasn't something I'd captured, not really. It was more like a gift from nature itself.

The maples stood amid a grove of cherry trees whose boughs wove an intricate canopy overhead. That tangled web led back down to gnarled trunks, beautifully contorted in ways that had inspired countless inkbrush scrolls and woodblock prints, corrugated skin flecked with amber knots of sap that glimmered like jewels when the sun hit them just right. Here and there I spotted coats of tiny mushrooms blooming on the bark, an unmistakable early sign of decay. As if to remind the old-timers of their dwindling lifespans, moss-covered stumps dotted the floor of the grove, remains of trees that had been culled after reaching their inevitable ends: graves of the sakura. Yet as I looked closer, I saw shoots sprouting from these supposedly dead places, too, tiny lives questing through carpets of moss toward the nourishing light. The raven had called my attention to this shrine, and the shrine to the trees, and the trees to their predecessors, and to the shoots rising from the loam—a subtle reminder of the cycle of life but also that death isn't truly an end. It is a beginning for other lives. Just like the new one I was trying to forge, after my mother died.

A warm sense of appreciation spread through my body, and tears filled my eyes. At that moment, I knew I wasn't alone, and never would be again.

In the traditional beliefs of my country, everything has a spirit. The heavens above, the ground below, the trees, the rocks, the rivers, the seas, even the words we speak. That is the fundamental essence of Shinto, the belief system native to the islands of Japan. The kami are the avatars of every aspect of the natural world, and Shinto is a method of interacting with them, which is to say a method for grappling with the never-ending cycles of life, birth, and death, and everything that came before, and everything that will come after.

That was the first time in my life I sensed the presence of the kami, the many-faced multitude of gods that once guided Japan. But wasn't that ancient history? Like most people, busy with studies and school, then work, I had never really paid them much mind. Now, I was beginning to realize, the kami were everywhere, if you knew where to look.

LEGEND HOLDS THAT THE ISLANDS OF JAPAN ARE HOME TO "yaoyorozu-no-kami," or "eight million kami." This idiom, widely used even today, is in fact poetic license, less a concrete accounting than an awed description of an uncountable multitude. Kami are invisible avatars of awesome forces beyond human control. They are the faces of a multifaceted complexity that would otherwise boggle the human imagination. And "eight million" is a gentle shorthand that suggests there's always room for more.

The title of this book has used a bit of poetic license, too: one name for a world of spirituality that offers countless potential journeys. The kami are but the beginning.

Eight million ways to happiness sounds like a tall order. Even more so if one treats eight million as an unfathomably large number. But "happiness and unhappiness can't be considered objectively," said the celebrated sumi-e ink artist Toko Shinoda when asked about the subject in 2020, at the age of 107. "One who abhorred the brush would feel nothing but torment in the life I have led. A thousand people will have a thousand different values as regards the matter." To Shinoda, happiness was a question of perspective. And there are as many of those as there are people alive, and people who have ever lived. An unfathomably large number indeed.

What is happiness? Some of the greatest Japanese minds of the past century have wrestled with the question. "The notion that one's goal in life is to be happy, that your own happiness is the goal?" asked anime director Hayao Miyazaki. "I just don't buy it." The author Yukio Mishima was even more ambivalent, declaring the contemplation of happiness a "risky matter." Others have taken a more pragmatic approach. In *Afternoon in the Islets of Langerhans*, the novelist Haruki Murakami suggests that happiness can be found in the minutiae: tearing into a freshly baked loaf of bread with one's hands, wearing a clean new shirt, or even the sight of neatly folded underwear in a drawer. Which happens to sound a lot like another purported path to happiness: Marie Kondo's cleaning magic.

As I stewed in misery over so much loss so quickly, I, too, questioned what happiness was. I recall a lunch with a mutual friend of the classmate who had passed away. "You're so lucky you can feel sadness over your mother's passing," she said. "You must have had such a happy life together." Perhaps she meant these words as comfort, but they twisted in me like a knife. "I envy you so much," she continued, before launching into a tirade about her own mother, offered, I suppose, as a foil to the happiness she imagined I'd experienced with mine.

Except: She knew nothing about my relationship with my mother. Nothing about how I'd struggled with her, how I'd craved her recognition even as I fumed over the way she compared me with my younger sister, constantly and inevitably unfavorably. Or the terrible fights my mother and I had had, the terrible words exchanged, words that haunted me even still. Maybe my friend had similar "mom problems." But there was a big difference between the two of us.

Her mother was still alive. I'd just buried mine, and there were no more conversations to be had.

In my fragile state, words could cut as deeply as any blade. My friend's clumsy projection of happiness onto my grief, no matter how well intentioned, only served to push solace even further away.

I continued walking in the park every day. Slowly, over days and weeks, I noticed my senses return. I started feeling the warmth of the sun again. I started noticing little things. The light dancing across the surface of the lake I circled on my walks. Calico koi fish nosing for food beneath floating islands of fallen maple leaves. Birds chattering in the canopy, sparrows, kingfishers, and the occasional squawk of a blue heron, soaring overhead like a pterodactyl. The trees, having long since shed their autumn hues, budding once again. All of it quietly but firmly reminding me that the park was filled with life.

Before I set foot in that shrine, I saw death as the period on the end of every story, my relationship with my mother's included. But the sakura grove reminded me how wrong I was. In full bloom, a sakura's beauty is breathtaking: twisted boughs disappearing beneath a gentle embrace of pink flowers as soft as clouds. Yet even at the spectacular peak of their full bloom, the first cherry petals begin to drift away from the branches, a few at first, then over the days to come, a rain that carpets the ground. Within a week, glory has come and gone. The sakura is a tree, but it is also a metaphor for the bittersweet impermanence of things. We treasure the cherry precisely because its beauty is as radiant as it is fleeting. It is a living poem that reminds us of ourselves.

My encounter with the sakura in the shrine, even dormant in the fall, reminded me of something when I needed it most. My mother was gone, but I lived on. I lived because of her. Her death wasn't an end; it was a baton being passed. I had a responsibility to run with it, to treasure the gift she had given me: myself. I can't say the realization made me happy; the wounds were still too fresh for that. But my brush with the kami kindled embers of gratitude within me, and that was a start.

I CALLED KAMI "GODS" ABOVE, BUT THAT WAS JUST SHORT-hand. The word *kami* resists easy interpretation—for Japanese people or otherwise. God—especially when written with that capital *G*—is so freighted with Western religious, political, and emotional baggage as to render it almost useless as a translation. Kami are kami, products of a thoroughly non-Judeo-Christian worldview.

In the eighteenth century, the philosopher Norinaga Motoori defined kami as "anything whatsoever that is outside the ordinary, that has superior and extraordinary power, provoking awe, but not exclusively, for they also encompass the wicked and the strange." More recently, the cultural anthropologist Dr. Kazuhiko Komatsu wrote that "the word 'kami' contains, whether negative or positive, all spiritual beings," in which he included spirits of the natural world, deities venerated at shrines and temples, yokai goblins, ghosts, and departed ancestors. Kami are the names people of old gave to the features of the world that astonish in their magnificence, or to forces that are deserving of respect or that they thought required some form of appeasement to keep in check.

I suspect that few Japanese have pondered what kami are at all, because kami are such an integral part of the landscape here, such a part of the fabric of daily life, that the concept of questioning them doesn't even arise. We use a verb, *matsuru*, to cover a huge variety of situations in which we interact with kami, ranging from quiet respect to communal services, from solo prayer to official deification and enshrinement. I have never been able to square the generally accepted translation of *pray*, which feels too vague for the huge spectrum of behaviors matsuru encompasses. Nor *worship* or *venerate*, which seem to me to invite biblical imagery of supplication and prostration. The difference between worship and matsuru feels like the difference between a digital on-off switch and an analog dial. We do venerate the kami, but they're part of everyday life, and we are surrounded by reminders of them: as big as a grand shrine or as small as a paper talisman of the sort many keep in their homes. The kami can't be seen, but they're always there. They are avatars of the forces at work in the natural world, big and small.

Hectic modern lives are filled with noise, literal and metaphoric. When you live a busy life, you naturally find yourself becoming the center of it—or in another sense, the top of it: You, Inc. It's lonely up there at the top, just you against the world, in a sea of troubles, with no cushion between yourself and the outrageous slings and arrows of fortune. Acknowledging the kami isn't a form of enlightenment or life-changing magic. It is like a pause, a reminder that you are part of a bigger web in which you play an important, but by no means solo, part.

After that experience in the park, I began reconnecting with my nation's spiritual traditions through a long, self-directed study of Shinto. This wasn't as easy as it sounds. For all its millennia of history, Shinto does not possess a sacred text, à la the Torah or Bible, or the sutras of Buddhism. Still, there are a great many books published on the topic in Japanese, and my newfound interest arrived with impeccable timing. In 2012, the largest Shinto organization in Japan, the Association of Shinto Shrines, inaugurated an official series of Shinto Cultural Examinations, designed to promote knowledge of domestic religious traditions among citizens. I dove into my studies, and I passed my certification the following year. All the while, I traveled throughout Japan visiting holy spots, to see these places, speak with locals, and learn about how we Japanese apply religious traditions in our daily lives, in ways conscious and not.

You have to understand what a jump this was for me.

Before my mother died, I didn't think of myself as religious. I still don't, not in any organized sense. I grew up in an average Japanese home in an average Tokyo suburb. I studied abroad, as many young Japanese did then, once in high school and later for university. I lived in America for a decade after, which is when I met the American man who would later become my husband. Those were fun years. The two of us built a small company that specialized in what was, in the nineties, an occupation so arcane that it didn't have a name yet: producing English translations of Japanese video games. Together we navigated the twin shoals of international marriages, with their inevitable cultural differences, and of going into business with one's spouse. Somehow, we made it work and carved out a niche for ourselves in what would soon prove to be a booming field known as localization.

We spent our days working with other people's ideas but yearned to create our own. In the first decade of the 2000s, that's exactly what we did. Together we wrote a series of illustrated guidebooks to Japanese folklore, produced in a fun "survival guide" format: one about yokai, which are monsters from myth; then a sequel for ninja, the subject of so much lore in their own right; and eventually a third, about yurei, the ghosts that have haunted Japan's nightmares from time immemorial.

Looking back now, I can see how these experiences were like a trail of breadcrumbs leading me to the heart of Japan's spiritual traditions. I first traveled to America on a home-stay program for the simple reason that I wanted to learn to speak English. But I quickly realized that language is more than just a tool. It is a product of its culture. Understanding, true understanding, requires more than simply opening a bilingual dictionary and swapping words.

One of my earliest conversations with my American host family sticks with me even today. My homestay family had a coffee-table book of Japanese calligraphy, and they asked if I could write like that, too. This was handwriting by true masters of the brush, work so exquisite that it was considered fine art by the Japanese and, if the book was any indication, by Westerners, too.

Of course, I couldn't write like this. Very, very few could. I tried to convey this. What I'd have said in Japanese was that my handwriting was too "kitanai," meaning messy, to even attempt calligraphy. I hastily consulted a pocket-size paperback Japanese-English dictionary for a translation. There it was.

"My writing is too . . . *dirty*!" I said with a satisfied smile on my face.

This really threw my homestay parents for a loop.

I'd fallen into a classic trap of translation: context. The word *kitanai* can indeed mean "dirty," as in the context of a dirty dish or shirt. But while *kitanai* can also be applied to writing in Japanese, *dirty* applied to writing in English evokes something completely different—something vulgar.

It took several back-and-forths, but they finally figured out what I was getting at.

"Hiroko, what you mean to say is 'my handwriting is too *poor.*'"

Now I was the one thrown for a loop. I'd been taught this word in school, but the only meaning I knew for it was someone without any money.

We eventually figured it out. It was an everyday sort of exchange, and I wouldn't be surprised if my homestay family had long since forgotten it. But I never did. It was my first lesson that context is everything.

After founding our company, we spent our days bridging

cultures, between mine and those of audiences abroad. And I started realizing that there was a lot of context missing, not of the linguistic but of the spiritual variety. Consumers knew Japan's characters, even to a degree its history and culture, from cartoons and games and all the other things we were translating for them. But when it came to spirituality, it was as if there were a big black hole. There wasn't much written about our ways, and the portrayals of them in Western fan circles or even mass media tended to be quite strange. And to be honest, I didn't think much about the spiritual side of Japan myself, not in any concrete way.

The irony is that while few Japanese identify as religious, my nation is something of a spiritual wonderland. There are many temples and shrines, of course, but also countless smaller stone effigies and memorials and statues of all sorts to be found, quietly sitting on city corners or countryside roads. Those smaller manifestations of spiritual traditions are really everywhere once you start looking for them, and I often did, even as a young girl. Whenever I found one of these little monuments, I'd always stop and check it out: the shapes, the weathered inscriptions, often too blurred by the decades to read. Who'd put it there, and why? I particularly liked the little "jizo" bodhisattva statues found so often along pathways and at crossings. They were like little children carved of stone, standing watch over their surroundings. Their rounded heads might be pitted by decades or centuries of weather, but they would inevitably be wearing a colorful hand-sewn cloth bib, crafted by some local who cared for them. If I saw a jizo, I'd be drawn as if by a magnet, pressing my palms together and bowing in greeting, even though I had no idea what they represented in a religious sense. Perhaps it was my sensing the tenderness with which someone tended to them, reminding me, even then as a little girl who didn't know much about the world, that there are good people out there. For if someone would lavish such attention on a such a small stone figure, they must be kindhearted indeed.

But I didn't think in such analytical terms back then. I saw nothing special about this, nothing different, really, than my exchanging pleasantries with someone I might pass on the street. There was nothing I'd have identified as religious about this attitude or behavior. I did it because it felt good, and right. As I grew up, I continued doing it. This wasn't what English speakers call belief or faith. Those words are declarative, definitive, binary: You have them or you don't. This wasn't like that. My feelings for these statues seemed to well from someplace deeper, borders uncertain, form diffuse, but no less powerful in its pull.

After my mother passed, I continued pressing my hands together whenever I'd find a jizo or happen across a shrine or a temple. But something was different. I began questioning the instinct. *Why am I doing this?* My mother and father hadn't taught me. Nobody had. Yet all of us did it—parents, friends, strangers. What did it mean? Which led to a question that lingered, like an itch I couldn't scratch: If I didn't get to the bottom of it, if I didn't use all the experiences I'd had and gifts I'd been given to try and explain it, who would?

I had an inkling that the same things that fascinated me about my nation's spiritual traditions might be interesting to people outside of Japan as well—even useful. I don't mean this in a missionary sense, of hoping those abroad take up Japanese faith practices. Rather, I hoped readers could take a page from us when it comes to spiritual thinking.

My mother's death in 2008 plunged me into an abyss. My

encounter with the raven proved a turning point. Thirteen years later, in 2021, I lost my father. This plunged me back into the depths again. But this time, something felt different. I realized that the time I'd spent reconnecting with my nation's spiritual traditions helped me re-center myself.

I believe that our way of interacting with the spiritual world represents more than just heritage. It's a living culture that can inspire beyond borders. Japan is an advanced nation that wholeheartedly embraces high-tech conveniences. It is home to some of the world's most advanced medical care, efficient transportation systems, and globally compelling entertainments, from *Animal Crossing* to *Dragon Ball Z*. Yet tiny shrines continue to thrive inside crowded metropolises, surrounded by towering skyscrapers—even, occasionally, scraping the sky themselves, perched on top of them. In cities and countryside, the holy sites of multiple faiths can be found side by side, often quietly sharing patches of the same sanctified real estate.

So many societies seem to treat religion as an all-or-nothing affair. *Are you or aren't you?* But when Japanese profess to have little in the way of faith, it is less a declaration of secularity than it is a testament to the way we seamlessly slip in and out of our spiritual traditions. Whether it is to help us make it through rough spots, navigate big life transitions, or simply brighten our day, we pick and choose among philosophies as needed.

A famous saying describes the Japanese as "born Shinto, married Christian, and buried Buddhist." In practice, things aren't that simple; Japan's population is large, roughly half that of the United States, and there is a huge amount of individual variation. No small number of people do pledge allegiance to specific faiths, domestic and imported, old and new. Nevertheless, to the vast majority of Japanese people, religion isn't dogma. It is an anchor for all the dramas of our secular lives: big moments such as births and weddings and funerals, and little everyday moments, such as how we express gratitude for food, or each other. This isn't about identity or ideology but spirituality as a practical tool: Which tradition or ritual works best in this particular life circumstance?

In a movingly written, bestselling book titled *Wintering*, the British writer Katherine May depicts her struggles to incorporate spiritual tools into her modern mindset. As she wrestles with the "desire to find life in the world around me, the trees and stones and bodies of water, the birds and mammals that enter my line of sight," she uses words such as *embarrassed* and *ashamed*. Such "atavistic" thinking, she continues, makes her feel as though she were "disingenuously hanging with the rationalists while I furtively seek the numinous." It reminded me of just how freighted spirituality can be in the West, how the rational and ethereal are competitors, their coexistence a paradox that must somehow be reconciled. Yet when May describes her "personal animism, hushed by my conscious but nurtured by my unconscious," she might well be describing the mindset underlying much of Japanese culture. Not an *either-or* but a *both*.

My sense is that ritual is inextricably linked with faith in the West—something that is, almost by definition, performed as part of an organized religious service. In Japan, this isn't necessarily the case. If the average person prays at a Shinto shrine, or bows to a Buddhist jizo statue, few observers in Japan would interpret it as a declaration of faith. They might be devout, but it's even more likely that they are simply demonstrating a gesture of affection and respect. In contrast to traditions where rituals are used as boundaries, here in Japan, rituals often serve to bond us together. It's tempting to call this "ritual without belief," but as we'll explore in more detail in the pages to come, *Belief*-with-a-capital-*B* is actually beside the point. That's what makes it so easy for us to partake in little rituals borrowed from a patchwork of different ideologies.

The pioneer of peace and conflict studies, Johan Galtung, calls the blending of worldviews and traditions the building of "a spiritual toolbox." Creating one can help recenter us, help buffer us against fate. Japan is no mystical Shangri-la: As a nation, we suffer terribly from unhappiness and isolation, so much so that the government actually took the dramatic step of appointing a Minister of Loneliness in 2021. But Japan's problems are not unique. They mirror those of advanced societies across the globe. That means our spiritual lifestyle, which makes room for both tradition and modernity, for the faith-based and the rational, is more than just a quirk of culture. It's a potential guide for anyone struggling with a profound sense of disconnection anywhere. No matter how bad things get, no matter how lonely we might feel, we are not victims or hermits, even when it seems the glow of a screen is our only company. We are part of a much bigger story, one constantly unfolding. We and the eight million kami around us.

....

PRECIOUS FEW BOOKS ARE DEVOTED TO THE TOPIC OF JAP-anese spirituality in English. Most tend to be very old, steeped in artistic abstraction, or highly academic. Way back in 1894, the Japanologist Lafcadio Hearn lamented how "little has been written in English about Shinto, which gives the least idea of what Shinto is." Not much has changed in the 120 years since. But for those who've dipped a toe into Marie Kondo's tidying philosophy, searched for their "ikigai" (inner passion), or indulged in the Japanese art of forest bathing (as, for instance, Hillary Clinton says she did to get over the trauma of losing the 2016 presidential race)—indeed, for anyone struggling to come to terms with a world that seems more and more confusing and alienating by the day—I believe the time is ripe for a book that explores spirituality the way Japanese experience it.

My sense is that the West tends to be freer in terms of society and more rigid in terms of religion. Japan, I've come to realize, is the opposite: a nation with a rigid society but a surprising flexibility in regard to religion. In the West, *religion* means embracing a single theology, often connected to a specific institution. It implies strict boundaries and identities. That specificity isn't something a majority of Japanese citizens seem inclined toward, which is why, in survey after survey, so many of us claim not to have any religion at all. Superficially, this would seem difficult to square with the sheer number of sacred sites that exist in Japan. Buddhist temples, for instance, are some of the nation's biggest domestic tourist draws. How to explain this seeming conundrum? There are many organized religions active in Japan, but in actual practice, many of our shared spiritual traditions are more like social customs masquerading as religious practices than they are expressions of faith. We perform them less as devotions than because they are simply *what is done, and always has been done.*

This often leads to misunderstandings. This is why Western journalists write of religion being "taboo" in Japan, while a Japanese government survey simultaneously reports that the nation's registered religious organizations claim almost 180 million followers—in a nation whose population is only 125 million. This is a testament to two things: one, that there is no taboo against spirituality in Japan, and two, that Japanese don't see the lines between theologies as impenetrable as those beyond our borders seem to. You can claim an affinity for multiple traditions at the same time.

This book is a personal journey, but it's also a cultural history, and, hopefully, a sort of road map. In the pages to come, I will lend you my perspective, as a cultural bridge between the East and West, to reveal truths about Japanese spirituality in ways few others can. The book's journey begins with the discovery of a long-forgotten, century-old diary, which leads me to hidden spiritual wellsprings that nourish so much of what people love about Japan, from craftsmanship to cleanliness. Together we will trek into the mountains with practitioners of Shugendo, learning how they make friends of monsters real and metaphorical, all in order to cultivate a positive outlook. We will hold hands through my parents' funerals to learn the power of curating one's spiritual practices. We will visit what is widely considered the scariest patch of ground in downtown Tokyo, and come face-to-face with Japan's most furious kami, who reminds us that all of our emotions, even the seemingly negative ones, have the power to heal. We will ascend to the stage as I learn the sacred dance of the Shinto shrine maiden from an elderly master, a performance art designed not for human audiences but for the kami themselves. And finally, in the farthest reaches of rural Japan, we will meet an itako shamaness, the last of her kind. She is a living embodiment of Japan's patchwork spirituality, harnessing folklore, local traditions, and aspects of Shinto, Buddhist, and Shugendo ritual to connect people with their loved ones in the hereafter. And then I will see if she might bridge the worlds of living and dead for me as well.

I struggled with how to explain my journey. The rationalist in me wanted a linear story. But I soon realized that wouldn't work. As living things, we may forge through time in a straight line, but our minds certainly don't work that way. In our thoughts, in our hearts, we are constantly flitting back and forth, ruminating on what came before, imagining the roads ahead. I've come to think of my grief in the form of a pond, deep in the forests of my mind. It is fed by a spring of tears. Sometimes they well up in a trickle, at other times, a flood. Sometimes it's easy to understand what triggered a deluge; other times, it's a mystery. Whenever I notice changes, I peer in, hoping to fathom why I am feeling what I am feeling. Just as in a real pond, I see myself reflected there. But unlike in real waters, I don't always see the me of the moment. More often than not, I see myself in the past, sometimes younger, sometimes older, always against the backdrops of the memories from those different ages. This book is like a series of glimpses into that pond of my heart.

By its end, I hope to give you a sense of spirituality the Japanese way—and to awaken you to the idea of a spiritual flexibility that can nourish you through life's inevitable ups and downs, wherever you might be, whether you possess a personal faith or not. We are all subject to many forces beyond our control, but we are also part of a bigger natural system that can fortify us, if we know how to plug into it. Japan's spiritual toolbox is filled with "adapters" to help make those connections. It is a philosophy that celebrates spiritual differences, a lifestyle where one can engage with numerous traditions rather than being compelled to identify with just one. This isn't seen as a compromise, because nothing is lost, only gained. And we are richer for it.

In closing, several caveats. The first is that while I do touch upon history ancient and modern, this book is not intended as a comprehensive overview of Japan's religious development. There are many excellent academic texts available on that topic, and I highly encourage those wanting a deeper dive to seek them out. I should also stress that religions are not static, and there is a constant evolution of beliefs and practices among the devout. The modern incarnations of Shinto, Buddhism, and Shugendo can be subdivided into a great many independent schools of thought. I personally hew to no particular sect, and neither does this book.

Which leads me to stress another key point. Japan's traditional beliefs are not evangelical. I am not a missionary, nor do I have aspirations of being anyone's guru. I don't claim to have any solutions to the world's problems. In the broadest strokes, I talk about reconnecting with nature, calming yourself so that you can cultivate a sense of gratitude, and re-centering yourself. But these are simply methods for settling heart and mind so that *you* can take the right action, whatever it might be. These aren't escapes from reality; they are mental tools to help you navigate it. Grounding yourself in this way can help you deal with the world, and the people in it, in the way that is best for you.

This book is simply the chronicle of my journey, my experience of finding another way of looking at the world. That said, I do not think it is a coincidence that I had my initial epiphany outdoors, in a park, surrounded by water and trees and life. Many of Japan's spiritual traditions are in effect ritualized forms of interacting with nature, to put you back in tune with nature's rhythms and "language." Consider the way of praying at a Shinto shrine, for instance. One approaches the altar, bows twice, claps twice, puts hands together in prayer, and then bows again. (There are variations, but that's the basic formula.) What is this process doing? In essence, the act of praying at a shrine compels us to go outdoors, to take a moment of silence, and to acknowledge that we are part of a greater system. But you don't need a shrine to do these things.

I have seen a man bowing in deep reverence to the waves crashing before him, on a beach on the island of Amami Oshima. There was nothing human-made around, only sand and stone and sea. This place is known for its typhoons, but the islanders are well aware that these fierce storms are part of the cycle of the seasons and nature as a whole, which provide them with their livelihoods. This is why they pray to the sea itself, the source of all their fortunes, and occasionally their suffering, too—a power greater than themselves.

When I am outdoors, whether in my garden, my local park, or hiking in the mountains, I always make sure to take a quiet moment—to stop, absorb the sounds, the sights, the scents, even the tactile feel of the things around me. When I do this, I feel as though I am listening to the world again. And time and again I have been surprised at the insights this practice reveals.

This book will take us to some far-flung places, and we'll meet a host of fascinating folks, some dwelling in our human world, others in realms beyond. But you don't need to know anything about Japan to benefit from the lessons I learned. These takeaways are applicable to everyone, everywhere. I hope that through reading about my experience, you'll see that forging your own spiritual path, however you personally choose to define it, doesn't mean forging ahead by yourself. The kami speak—not in words but in quiet codes that are everywhere, if you know how to look and listen for them. I promise that if you open your heart to those messages, you'll realize, like I did, that you're never truly alone.

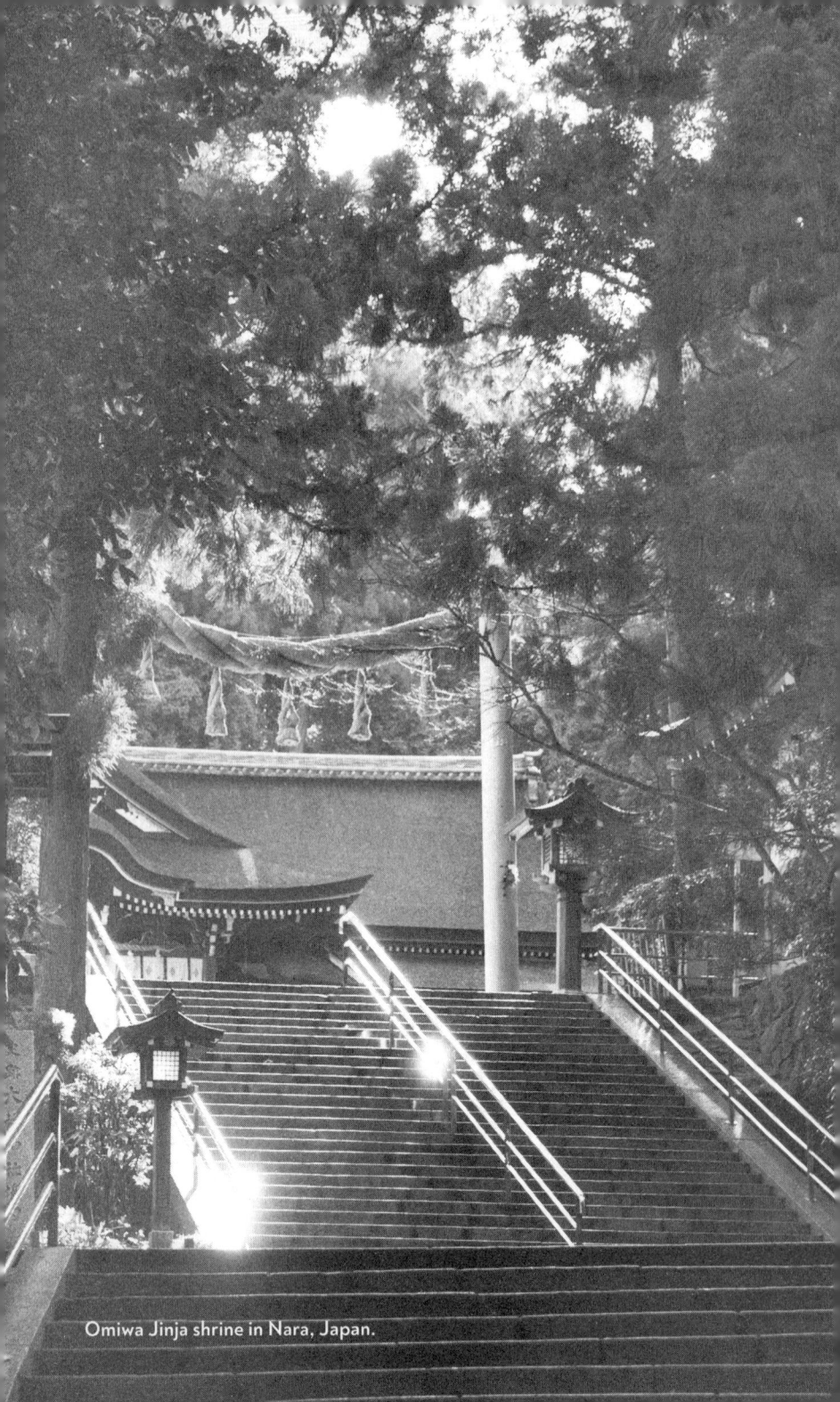

Omiwa Jinja shrine in Nara, Japan.

Part One

AWAKENING: EIGHT MILLION KAMI

CHAPTER I

The Invisibles: Shinto

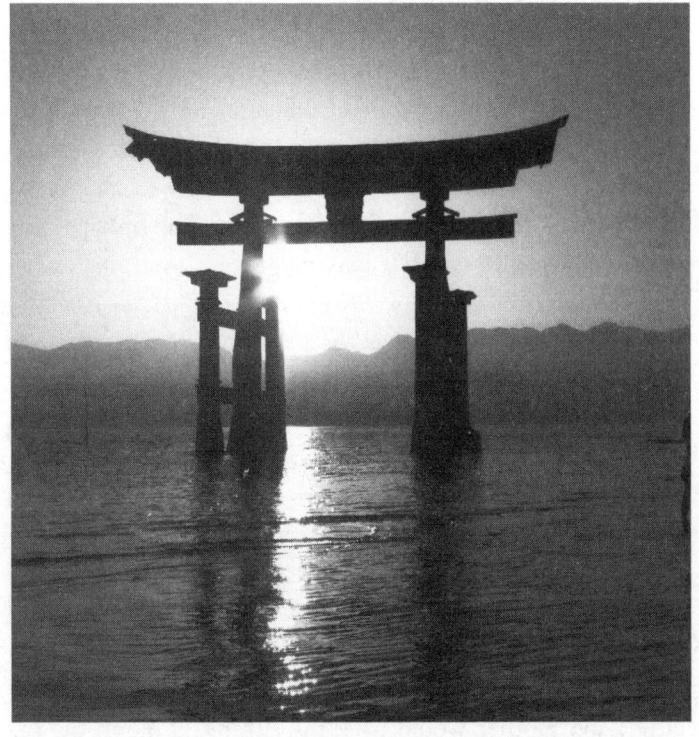

Itsukushima Jinja shrine in Hiroshima.

*That intimate sense of relation between the visible
and invisible worlds . . . is the special religious
characteristic of Japan.*

—Lafcadio Hearn, *Kokoro*, 1895

Ever since I was a little girl, I have liked to press my palms together in contemplation. Nobody showed me how to do this. Nor did I have any concept of prayer as a ritual. My parents weren't particularly religious, nor was anyone else in my tiny circle of family, friends, and schoolmates. I don't remember when, exactly, I tried it for the first time. But an early memory suggests that communicating with invisible people came naturally to me. At the age of about six, I invented a little game. The only participant was myself. I called it playing grave.

Lest you think I grew up among the *Addams Family*, I should explain a few things. As in many Asian cultures, in Japan it's common to maintain a family gravesite and visit several times a year, cleaning the stones, burning incense as an offering, and sharing stories about your loved ones. To us, visiting a cemetery isn't a macabre or even necessarily a sad occasion. And in my case, my paternal grandparents and my maternal grandmother died before I was born; my mother's father passed when I was just four. I have many pleasant memories of visiting his and my grandmother's grave. They were buried in a leafy suburb on the west side of Tokyo. My father and mother would pack my sister and me in the car for the hour-long drive to the memorial park, where we'd meet aunts, uncles, and cousins. First we would all pitch in to scrub moss and grime off the family marker: a squared obelisk of smooth granite standing about three feet high, inscribed with kanji, characters I could then barely read. Next, the grown-ups would place small bouquets of chrysanthemums and light sticks of incense, and we would lower our heads in silent prayer as the smoky perfume swirled around us. Then came the fun: a leisurely picnic lunch under the sakura trees, adults gossiping about adult things while we young ones darted off to play badminton. Even today, decades later, cherry blossoms conjure up dormant memories of those long-ago graveside gatherings. The taste of my mother's bento boxes: rice balls with tart pickled plum, the sweet softness of tamago-yaki omelets. The smell of wet stone and of freshly cut lawn, kicked up by my tiny legs running for, and usually missing, the shuttlecock.

I didn't get to experience growing up with a grandpa and grandma in my life. When you're a kid who doesn't have grandparents yourself, you sense just how much other kids talk about theirs—especially after a holiday.

"We took the bullet train to see my grandparents!"

"Grandma took me to the beach!"

"My grandpa gave me otoshi-dama," cash-filled envelopes doled out by relatives to kids at New Year's.

All of which was inevitably followed by others asking, "Oh yeah? How much did ya get?" and finally, once they'd exhausted their comparisons, the dreaded ". . . So how about *you*?"

My answer, of course, was "nothing." Every time I found myself entangled in this kind of conversation, the same thoughts ricocheted through my head: *I don't have grandparents. I never did.* I said this outright the first few times I was asked, but this would so obviously quash the mood that I quickly learned not to say anything at all. I'd shake my head and smile shyly and hope the focus shifted quickly, as it always did with kids. But the truth was that their stories weighed on my heart.

"Playing grave" emerged spontaneously one sunny suburban Tokyo afternoon. My mother was hanging laundry on the second-floor balcony. My baby sister was down for her nap, so there was nobody to play with. Wandering the house in my boredom, I found an empty shoebox on my father's side of their bed. It was brand-new, and shiny white. I sat down next to it, opened the lid, and lifted it up to examine. This stirred something in my six-year-old mind, and I was hit with an epiphany: "It's a grave!"

I carried the empty box outside and set it down on the opposite end of the balcony from where my mother was working. Then I took out a pencil and an orange paper flower I had found in my parents' closet, a poppy made of yellow paper folded and twisted over a piece of wire. I placed the bottom of the shoebox upside down in front of me like a table. On the lid, I used the pencil to carefully print *grandpa and grandma's grave*. It was an innocent, generic epitaph. No names, no specification of maternal or paternal; in my young mind, grandparents were grandparents, regardless of which side of the family they came from. Then I stood the lid up vertically along the side of the box. Finally, I laid the orange flower atop the makeshift altar.

There it was. My grandparents' grave. Proud of my handiwork, I put my hands together and closed my eyes, just as I'd seen my family and relatives do whenever we visited our family plot.

"What on earth are you doing?" came my mother's voice from behind.

"Playing grave," I replied without missing a beat. "You can pray here, too, if you want."

"No, thanks," she replied. Her face was a mask of studied indifference.

The problem with my ad hoc grave play was that there wasn't much to actually do; once you crouched down and pressed your palms together in silence, that was pretty much it. I quickly grew bored, and even felt a little silly. So I disassembled my grandparents' grave and put it away. I wonder what my father must have thought when he found his shoebox newly decorated with a generic epitaph penciled in a child's hand.

I laugh to myself whenever I remember this moment. What a strange child. My mother must have really wondered what was going on in my head. But over the years, as I've dusted off the memory from time to time, I've come to feel that it was about more than simply child's play. That it was telling me something, something important. I was, in effect, creating a space where I could mimic and experiment with Japanese traditions of communicating with invisible people.

With no memories of spending time together with my grandparents, I didn't have any concept of having lost them. My sadness wasn't caused by their death. It wasn't the anguish of loss but the disconcerting emptiness of something never having been there. All my friends seemed to have grandparents who cherished them. I didn't. So I did the next best thing: I imagined them. How they would play with me. How it would feel to hold their hands. Because I'd never met them, their faces were always blurred out in these fantasies. But in those moments they were glowing with an aura of love and kindness. In my mind they were like what a Westerner might call guardian angels. And on that one day when I was six, the fantasy crossed over into reality when I tried to reach out to them using nothing more than a pencil, a flower, and a new shoebox.

In his aptly titled 1894 book *Glimpses of Unfamiliar Japan*, Lafcadio Hearn noted that "in Japan there are two forms of the Religion of the Dead—that which belongs to Shinto and that which belongs to Buddhism." He was one of the first foreign visitors to pick up on differences in the ways death was handled between Buddhism, the religion imported to Japan from India by way of China and Korea some fourteen centuries ago, and Shinto, the native beliefs with a much longer lineage in Japan. Today, Japan's funeral traditions are almost entirely Buddhist in nature, and my game of pretend unconsciously incorporated motifs from my family visits to my grandparents' grave: the headstone inscribed with the names of the departed, the placing of the flowers, the prayers, the incense, all of it intended to ease their transition into the afterlife, all of it Buddhist in origin. At the time, I didn't think about things in those terms, of course. I wasn't even really conscious of the concept of religion, let alone ritual. All I wanted, hungered for, was contact. Contact with something I couldn't sense or see but knew, somehow, was there, something that I loved and that loved me. Years later I'd realize: Imbuing the invisible with a spiritual presence represented something altogether different from funerals, or from Buddhism. It was the fundamental essence of Shinto.

Shinto, written with characters meaning "The Way of Kami," is the name for the native spiritual beliefs of Japan. You'll note I said *spiritual* rather than *religious*. The reasons for my reluctance to use the *R* word will become more apparent later on, but I can tell you this much now: Growing up, we never heard about Shinto in class, we never went to the equivalent of a Sunday school. We went to shrines mostly as a sightseeing habit, saying, *Well, we're in Kyoto— maybe we should check out so-and-so shrine.* I doubt any among our friends and family could have articulated in any concrete detail what Shinto meant to us personally, let alone historically or culturally.

Yet we absorbed aspects of Shinto nonetheless, as if through osmosis. I remember a fad for colorful "omamori" in my all-girls high school. They are charms that are sold at shrines, made of cloth embroidered with glimmery lamé thread, with cord toggles that allow them to be hung on things for luck. There are many kinds: talismans for safe births, for safe travel, for successful studies, for finding a partner in marriage. All sorts of things. They aren't substitutes for caution or hard work. But no matter how hard you study or carefully you navigate traffic, accidents can happen. They are hopes for things to go well, and an admission that we can't control everything. Omamori are like packaged wishes.

But that's my grown-up hindsight talking. When we were girls, none of us treated omamori as sacraments. We simply loved them for their kawaii cute factor, with their embroidery and colors and beautifully knotted cords. We wore uniforms throughout middle and high school, dark blue blazers and skirts. The skirts fastened on one side, and we would hang an omamori from an open buttonhole as a decoration. Looking back, I guess that was a way for us to express a little individuality. Omamori were cute and colorful enough to catch attention, yet not so much so that they would trigger a dress-code infraction. Everyone wore different kinds, some received as gifts from family or friends, others purchased for their fortunes: charms for academic success, safety in commuting to school, or even just luck in general. I wore several over the years, but tellingly, I can't remember what specific protection any of them were supposed to confer. All I can remember is my favorite, which I bought on a school trip to Kyoto. A few girlfriends and I went to a shrine in Arashiyama, where we bought omamori featuring embroidered images of a beautiful lady-in-waiting in a kimono, a scene from *The Tale of Genji*. To me, omamori are like Shinto in a nutshell. They are quiet reminders of the forces out there beyond our control—and they're also simply nice to look at.

So we went to shrines and carried amulets, but none of us ever actually spoke of Shinto. One of the reasons for this was that the imperial government co-opted Shinto in the long lead-up to World War II, incorporating it into a colonialist ideology. Today, academics call it State Shinto. It ended abruptly with the arrival of the American occupiers in 1945, who rewrote our constitution to strictly separate church and state. Teachers in particular took this secular mandate very seriously.

But there is another, even bigger reason, I think. Shinto was always just *there*. And in many ways, this is how it always had been. Shinto didn't even get a name until well after the arrival of Buddhism in the sixth century. Until that point, there wasn't anything with which to compare it—it just *was*. I think this might well be the most fundamental aspect of Shinto. It isn't flashy or pushy. It doesn't call attention to itself. It's always in the background, existing patiently, waiting to be discovered—as I had, in the park with the raven and the shrine.

I don't think it's any coincidence that the spiritual journey that began after my mother's death led me to these native beliefs first. It is like a spiritual substrate for everything that came after, the foundation of so much of Japanese culture as a whole. I didn't consider myself Shinto then, and I don't consider myself to be Shinto now. But none of that matters. When you visit a shrine, you don't have to believe or disbelieve. You don't have to swear any kind of loyalty, or refuse any affiliations. That inclusivity, without any obligation other than showing commonsense respect, energized my explorations.

Shinto has no holy book, no scripture, no sermons, no evangelism. This is precisely what can make it so difficult to explain to those not raised here—because we would have equal difficulty explaining it to ourselves. When I started to reconnect with Shinto in a more serious way after my mother's death, I struggled with where to begin.

What helped me were stories. Stories that can be interpreted in many different ways, about the deities we call kami—kami that often behave a whole lot like people.

Let me tell you about the first of them.

EVERYTHING BEGINS, OF COURSE, AT THE BEGINNING: THE genesis of the heavens, the coalescing of the Earth out of the primordial void, and the creation of the islands of Japan by a pair of kami. One, Izanaki, was male; the other, Izanami, was female. Next, they invented sex. From her womb Izanami bore a multitude of kami, one after the other. The first to arrive was the kami of ambition: a symbol of commitment to their task. The very last to emerge was the kami of fire.

It burned Izanami terribly, mortally. In her death throes she vomited, producing a kami of mining and a kami of minerals. As she released her bladder and bowels, more kami sprang into existence: a pair of water kami from her urine, and the kami of soil and clay from her feces.

I should mention that all of this was news to me when I first decided to read the *Kojiki*. Translated as *Records of Ancient Matters*, it is Japan's first book, composed in 712 CE on commission from the emperor. It retells local legends already centuries old at the time, dispatches from a prehistory in which the membrane between the visible and invisible was thinner, and we saw spirits everywhere: in plants, animals, natural phenomena, even the very terrain itself. By respecting and venerating these presences as divine spiritual beings, inhabitants of the Japanese archipelago had always positioned themselves as part of something much bigger: a universal, natural order. This worldview is called animism, and it is the fundamental concept underpinning the traditional Japanese system of beliefs.

I turned to the *Kojiki* simply because, after my experience at the shrine in the wake of my mother's death, it seemed a natural place to start. Every Japanese learns about the existence of the *Kojiki* in school, but that's about the extent of it. The archaic text is hard to read, for one thing, and as I said, the constitution forbids public schools from engaging in religious education. Before reading it, what few kami names I did know came mainly from vague memories of explanations posted outside shrines, plaques detailing which or another of the kami were venerated there. Whenever I prayed at a shrine, it was always to a generalized kami-sama, or "honored kami," plural, multiple, rather than singling out any one in particular. I suspect the same is true for most Japanese. Not unlike how I prayed to my grandparents, plural, when I played grave as a little girl.

When I first read of Izanami's death, I really struggled with the idea of bodily functions producing kami. At first glance it seemed puerile, even vulgar. In my mind, I knew it wasn't meant this way. Japan was an agrarian nation, its people much more in touch with the earthier sides of life and death than we modern folk. Things we perceive as taboo today were handled regularly by them in the course of making a living: excrement as fertilizer, for example. I had to come to grips with the idea that the things that come out of our bodies might have had different values to them. And that led to an even bigger realization. At no point in the *Kojiki* are the kami ever explicitly described as human. Their appearances are described only in the broadest of strokes—beautiful, or ugly, for instance. But even here our human values fail. We consider "beautiful" good and "ugly" bad. But one of the most beautiful female kami, an avatar of cherry blossoms, symbolizes a fleeting life, while one of the ugliest, her sister the kami of rock and stone, is an avatar for the only meaningful currencies of the human condition: health and longevity.

Kami are things unseen, or rather, that cannot be seen. Their personification is a metaphor, a tool to help us understand forces unfathomable to our human minds. Izanami's end wasn't about filth at all. It was a story about a creator who died in the course of creation, one so divine that literally every part of her, and everything she produced, had profound meaning. Which is, in a sense, true of us all. We are nourished by what others before us have left behind, and in turn nourish others with the things we leave behind.

....

AFTER MY MOTHER DIED, MY SISTER AND I TOOK CARE OF TI-dying up her belongings. My father remained too sunk in his own grief to deal with them, and we wanted to help in any way we could. In the years before her passing, my mother had lost her ability to navigate stairs, and so she and my father had taken to sleeping in what had been the living room, with her on a rented orthopedic hospital bed. Now that she was gone, it was time to return it. The sight of the empty bed weighed heavily on all of us, my father most of all.

Beneath the bed had been placed several plastic drawers for supplies. When my sister cleaned them out, she found something unexpected. At the very back, behind folded piles of pajamas and such, was an old envelope. Inside it was a small stack of photographs, sepia-toned, spotted from age. We'd never seen any of them before—even my father. How had they gotten in there?

One of them showed a family sitting on the engawa, the low porch of a traditional home. In back kneeled a serious-faced older man in a dark hakama robe, with balding pate and round glasses. To his side were a trio of young women in kimonos, one holding an infant. In front of them sat a gaggle of three little girls, short legs dangling outside the house. There was no mistaking the one in the center of the frame, in a pinafore dress and clutching a stuffed animal: She was obviously my mother. I flipped it over. It was marked 1937. She would have been four years old. It was the first photo I had ever seen of her as a child, and it stirred complicated emotions inside me. She had been a little girl once, just as I had. Of course I'd known that intellectually, but here in my hand was undeniable proof. My mother kept these photos close to her heart. Even to the end.

After much discussion over several phone calls with extended family members, we pieced it together. That was my mother, of course, and her sisters, their mother, and two aunts. The older gentleman was my great-grandfather, whose house they were visiting on some long-ago get-together.

I'd known of his existence because my great-aunt, who lived near us and with whom I'd spent a lot of time growing up, was also in that faded photograph. She had passed away in 2000 but had spoken of him often. He was a great man, she'd always said. He was a scientist who had done great things.

That sent me online to look for more information. I was surprised to discover that my great-grandfather had his own Wikipedia page. I learned from it that he wasn't only a scientist. He was a mountaineer, and a serious one, the first director of the Japanese Alpine Club, the first of its kind in Asia. But there was an even bigger surprise to come, several years later.

My cousin was cleaning out his house in preparations to renovate, and stumbled across a wooden box in my great-aunt's possessions. Inside were three old books, handbound and handwritten in that beautifully precise calligraphy that one could attain only from a lifetime of writing with brush and ink rather than a computer. These were diaries, my great-grandfather's records of his alpine expeditions. Dense columns of text filled the vertically ruled pages, punctuated here and there by inkbrush drawings of climbing routes or particularly striking scenery. The first entry was dated 1899. It focused on his visit to a place called Mount Sanjo-gatake.

My eyes widened. I had been there myself. It is considered one of Japan's holiest peaks and is the center of a spiritual tradition called Shugendo, a mixture of Shinto and Buddhist and other philosophies. This esoteric school of mountain worshippers fascinated me, because I've always loved mountains, too. And as my eyes raced over the page, as quickly as I was able to process the archaic handwritten text, I saw that he had walked where I had walked, seen what I had seen. There was a sketch of a view I immediately recognized, because I had stood there myself, 120 years after he had. I knew it intimately, because I used a photo I'd taken there for the background of my computer desktop. Seeing my grandfather's rendition made me feel as though I were looking through his eyes for a moment. It gave me goose bumps.

He was a man of modernity, a scientist and alpinist, yet had sought out these spiritual experiences and written about them. We were on parallel journeys, walking together, my footsteps in his, separated only by time. We could never speak, for he had died long before I was ever born. But he had left me his thoughts in these pages. I was still processing the loss of my mother, and struggling to contextualize the things I was seeing on my own explorations. My great-grandfather's diaries felt as though the messages I'd sent "playing grave" so long ago had finally returned a response.

"The Nineteenth Century is over, and dawn has broken over the Twentieth," he wrote at the beginning of the third volume, in an entry dated January 1901. "Times have changed, and I hope I have changed with them, yet my habits remain ingrained: travel and mountaineering. An infinity of years stretch ahead, yet I have but a handful of decades left. I hope I can write about even more mountains, and as I look at the blank sheafs before me, I am filled with hope of finding new scenery, new people, and to make a fresh start for myself. I hope what I am now isn't what I was in the years previous."

My great-grandfather's words, put to paper 120 years ago, reminded me of something that I learned in my studies: tokowaka. It's a Shinto term that isn't widely used in daily speech, but is written with characters meaning "forever young." At first glance this might sound like a trite celebration of youth. But tokowaka is about much more than that. It's about remaining true to yourself even as the times change around you. It tells us that the way to stay young isn't by embracing the past but rather in having the courage to change. I think this is what he meant by *I hope what I am now isn't what I was.*

Let me explain with a famous example from Japanese architecture. The Grand Shrine of Ise is dedicated to Amaterasu, the kami of the sun. Built entirely of fragrant Japanese cypress in a style unchanged from its founding 1,300 years ago, it represents one of Japan's most striking pieces of spiritual architecture. "The beauty of Ise, from my first glimpse of the Isuzu River and the magnificent trees, quite overwhelmed me," wrote the Japanologist Donald Keene of his first visit, in 1953. "I had visited other Shinto shrines, but the experience here seemed totally different because of the special, holy atmosphere."

The grand shrine is beautiful, but that isn't the reason for its fame. The day Keene visited was special indeed: It was the end of the "Shikinen Sengu." This is a ritual in which the entire shrine is dismantled, rebuilt, and re-unveiled to the public every twenty years. Shrines, especially grand ones like Ise, cost a lot of money to build. They are meticulously cleaned and maintained. It might seem strange, even wasteful, to do this to a perfectly usable structure. But Shikinen Sengu is no demolition. It is a rejuvenation, and one that takes place slowly, over many years. As parts of the building are removed and replaced, the old pieces are donated to other shrines throughout Japan so that they might renovate themselves. And the reconstruction nourishes the skill sets of carpenters and craftspeople, so that the old production techniques are never lost. The Grand Shrine of Ise has been taken apart and rebuilt every twenty years for well over a millennium. *Times have changed*, to paraphrase my great-grandfather, *but habits remain ingrained.* Tokowaka isn't a pursuit of youth at all; it is about striving to keep a youthful mindset in the face of the relentless march of time. It teaches us the power of making a fresh start, at regular intervals.

The discovery of those photos and diaries, left by my mother and great-grandfather, certainly felt like someone or something telling me to make a fresh start. And it also reminded me how fresh starts are at the root of so much of Japanese culture. It's at the heart of our cleaning customs, such as the osoji, the great cleanings families traditionally carried out at year's end, for the obvious reasons of tidying up but also as a kind of mental reset for the new year to come. Shinto purification rituals are designed to spiritu- ally "disinfect" you to make you more presentable to the kami before praying at a shrine, but they're also designed to reinvigorate you, personally, "sweeping away" negative feelings—anger, bad memories, shame, anything holding you down—in hopes of helping you refresh yourself.

In fact, one of Japan's foundational myths is about a reset, of sorts. Perhaps the greatest reset of all. It's about a day the sun decided not to come up. And within this story can be found all the reasons why Shinto shrines look the way they do, and how we interact with them today.

LONG, LONG AGO, THE KAMI DWELLED IN THE HIGH PLAINS of the heavens. Among them were Amaterasu and her youn- ger brother Susano'o. They were polar opposites: She was the kami of the sun, a cultivator of beauty and order, and Susano'o was a brutish, unpredictable agent of chaos. Susano'o continually provoked his sister, ransacking her palace's rice fields, defiling her living quarters, terrorizing her hand-maidens. Again and again, the kindhearted Amaterasu forgave him. But everyone has their breaking point, and like many younger brothers, Susano'o was a master at finding his sister's. Waiting for a quiet moment when Amaterasu watched her maidens weaving cloth, Susano'o leapt atop her palace, ripped open the roof, and hurled the skinned corpse of a horse through the opening into the room below.

Enough was enough. Amaterasu resolved to leave the world, never to return. She retreated into a heavenly rock cave, then sealed the entrance with a giant boulder. As a result, the entire world went dark, for Amaterasu's absence deprived it of light. Total darkness was a calamity. Crops could not grow. Famine and sickness spread across the land.

This would not do. The eight million kami gathered around the cave, trying all sorts of things to try and lure Amaterasu out. One gathered mythical birds so that their song might fill the air. Another created a mirror, then yet another created long strings of magatama, curved beads carved from semiprecious stone. These were hung from the branches of an uprooted sakaki tree as an offering. Another kami brought a deer bone to use in bone divination fortune-telling. Another recited a ceremonial chant. Then a female kami carried a bucket over to the sealed entrance of the cave, flipped it over into a makeshift stage, climbed atop it, and began to dance.

This dance performance caused a great deal of mirth among the countless kami. The crowd grew boisterous, laughing in glee—a real party. Amaterasu heard the commotion. She opened the stone door just a crack. "I have plunged the world into darkness. Yet all of you are playing and laughing. Why?"

The dancer answered. "We have found an even higher and more honorable kami than you, my lady, and we celebrate her here."

This perplexed the Sun Goddess, who wondered who this newcomer might be. Two kami rushed up bearing the mirror.

"There she is!" they cried. "Why don't you see her for yourself?"

Intrigued by her own reflection, Amaterasu peeked out of the crack in the door for a better look. As her hand emerged, another kami took it and guided her out of the cave. The assembled quickly stretched a braided rope behind her, blocking any return inside.

The Sun Goddess had returned, and the world brightened once again.

....

THIS STORY IS ONE OF THE ORIGIN STORIES OF SHINTO. IT IS also a blueprint for how a shrine is constructed. *Tori'i* means a Shinto gate, but it is written with characters meaning "bird's roost," a call back to the mythical birds that the kami used to try and lure Amaterasu out of hiding. Larger shrines often have a structure called a kagura-den, a hall for dancing— just as the female kami danced for her fellow deities. The braided shimenawa that denote sacred spots within shrine grounds are the descendants of the rope strung by the kami to guide Amaterasu out of the cave. Within a shrine's sanctum, you might catch sight of a priest reciting a ritual chant. And most deep inside, the physical avatar of a particular shrine's kami will often (not always, but often) be shielded from sight by a mirror, just like the one the kami used to lure Amaterasu out of hiding so long ago.

Shrines come in all shapes and sizes. Some are humble

little boxes tucked into a street corner or a park, like the one I encountered during my walks after my mother's passing. Others are larger structures. Still others are surrounded by entire campuses of outbuildings. A few are so splendid that they have become major international tourist destinations in their own right. But things didn't start out this way. In times of old, long before the first jinja was ever erected, our ancestors focused their spiritual energies on the terrain surrounding them, and in particular on natural rock formations. Today we call these ancient holy spots iwakura.

It's written with the characters for "rock-seat," for ancient Japanese believed that kami descended from their realm to dwell in stones. Why stones? Iwao Oba, a professor of Shinto archaeology, has suggested a simple reason. Trees rot and soil erodes, but rocks retain their shapes for very long periods of time. Perhaps this is why people of old saw in them a metaphor for stability—recall that the kami of stone is also the kami of longevity.

Old iwakura can still be found throughout Japan, if you know where to look. And after starting to study Shinto, I very much wanted to look. Iwakura really "sang" to me, as someone who loved mountains and spiritual traditions both.

For the first iwakura I visited, in those early months of reading up on Shinto history and lore, I picked one of the most famous, located in the foothills of Mount Kamikura, in Wakayama Prefecture.

Millennia ago, says the *Kojiki*, Mount Kamikura is where a legendary warrior met a three-legged spirit-raven. It served as his guide on a perilous journey. At the end of the journey, the warrior became Jimmu, the mythical first emperor of Japan. On the slopes of Kamikura can be found an iwakura that locals call Gotobiki-iwa: Toad Rock. It sounds cute, almost like a mascot character. But it is in fact one of the nation's largest and most impressive iwakura. This is a place where ancient and modern spiritual traditions entwine, where we can brush fingertips with those threads as they spool from distant past into far future.

To get to Toad Rock, one must navigate a serpentine staircase of 538 rough-hewn stone steps that ascend through a fragrant cedar forest. These steps were originally the gift of a shogun, Minamoto-no-Yoritomo, in the twelfth century. They're still being used today, almost a thousand years later. When I first huffed and puffed up that ancient staircase, I had to watch my feet. Over the centuries, soft carpets of moss and lichen had enveloped the stones, and a light rain made things slippery. But the rain also eased my efforts in a way. Every time I pressed a boot into that spongy surface and lifted it, the scent of the forest rose around me, a natural form of aromatherapy no perfume could hope to match.

Midway up, I noticed a small creek trickling down the mountainside. The flow was so gentle, it was almost still, but the water was far too clear and clean to be stagnant. I peered closer and was startled to see something peering back: a Japanese firebelly newt. Its pebbly black skin blended in so perfectly with the leaves and loam of the creek bed, making it almost invisible. But when it caught sight of my face, it tucked in its tiny feet and jetted off with a flick of its body, revealing a flash of the blazing crimson underbelly that gives the critters their common name. It reminded me of something my husband had once told me. He'd been so excited when we first encountered a newt when we were hiking together, years back. He and his family had raised them as pets when he was growing up in the States. They'd purchased them from pet stores; he'd never seen one in the wild before. They were delicate creatures, he told me, and they could thrive only in the cleanest of water. Clean water means clean soil, healthy plants and trees, and an entire, balanced ecosystem. The little newt suggested an environment healthy enough to support such small and sensitive lives.

I continued climbing the long staircase. Finally, I rounded the last corner. As the Gotobiki-iwa came into view, all I could think was: *Whoa.* In a way, that "whoa" *is* Shinto: *This place is special. This place is worthy of respect.* At thirty-six feet tall, the boulder is the height of a three-story building— and another twenty-six feet around. Perched high on this hillside like a sentinel, it watches over the city and ocean below. It's easy to understand why people of old saw this as a holy place. A modern shrine had been constructed here to mark it now; its crimson woodwork reminded me of that newt down trail. Old and new, side by side.

Gotobiki-iwa is, in one way of thinking, just a big rock. But it also serves as the waystation on a journey: from the "normal world" outside, through that delicate forest ecosystem, to this long-venerated spot and back again. That made this giant stone something like an ambassador. It couldn't speak, of course, but its silence was not impassive. Toad Rock was surrounded by many lives, ranging from tiny creatures to majestic cedars. No, this was more than a boulder. It was a model, a microcosm, a reminder that each of our existences is a "rock" surrounded by a much bigger system of countless lives with whom we interact.

Many millennia have passed since the distant ancestors of modern Japanese began venerating stones as iwakura. This early period of what might be called proto-Shinto is shrouded in mystery: We aren't sure what these holy people looked like, how they were seen by their communities, or what their rituals consisted of. Some hints can be found, however, on Okinoshima, whose name literally means "island of the far sea," but which might better be termed the Island of the Kami.

Thirty-seven miles off the coast of Kyushu, near the city of Fukuoka, Okinoshima lives up to its name. It sits in a patch of ocean known as Genkai-nada, "the rough seas of the north." Powerful currents, churning waves, and hidden shoals make this one of the most abundant fishing grounds in Japan. But they also make it one of the region's most dangerous waterways, and maps of the area are dotted with the sites of shipwrecks. Okinoshima is a mysterious place today; it must have been even more so long ago. Perhaps this is why the ancients repeatedly ventured forth to hold protective rituals there. Seen from a distance, the island's silhouette rises out of a blue haze like a fin. Up close, craggy cliffs ring a plateau covered in primeval forest; deep within stands a simple, wooden Shinto shrine—what must be the single least-visited in all of Japan.

The residents of the nearest port town, to which Okinoshima officially belongs, have long restricted access to the sacred island. For many years, only two hundred were permitted to visit just once annually on a chartered ferry, but even then they were formally requested never to speak of what they had seen there. And they were all men. Okinoshima has always been off-limits to women. The reasons for this are not clear but probably represent a vestige of now-archaic Shinto beliefs treating blood, and thus menstruation, as impurities.

The ancients didn't limit themselves to rocks. They believed kami resided in all sorts of terrain; trees, waterfalls, and mountains were all treated as potential "seats." There are holy grounds that consist of just a tori'i gate standing in front of a mountain. No building at all, because what's being venerated is nature itself. A shrine is simply a receptacle for the kami. They don't "live" in any structure created by human hands, any more than the people we communicate with by telephones live inside them. Shrines are tools for communication, temporary residences through which the divine might descend if we coax them into bestowing upon us their presence. Even the grandest shrine is, essentially, empty inside.

Lafcadio Hearn learned this in the spring of 1890. He had recently arrived in Yokohama as a correspondent for *Harper's Magazine*, charged with gathering local color for a readership hungry for dispatches from the exotic Orient. One day not long after his arrival, Hearn paid a local guide to take him on a tour of local holy spots.

The guide brought Hearn to a flight of stone steps, the steepest and loftiest the journalist had ever seen. He began to climb. At the top, winded and exhausted from his exertion, Hearn discovered an old shrine. It was a small wooden building, bedraggled gray by the elements—"chill even in the sun, bleak, and desolate, as if no prayer had been uttered in it for a hundred years." But a paper screen clattered open, and an elderly priest emerged from within. Hearn was likely the first foreign person the old man had ever seen. Still, he beckoned the strange new visitor inside. So it was that the journalist found himself among the very first Westerners to penetrate the heart of a Shinto sanctum.

"I reach the altar, gropingly, unable yet to distinguish forms clearly," he writes in the *Glimpses of Unfamiliar Japan*. "But the priest, sliding back screen after screen, pours in light upon the gilded brasses and the inscriptions; and I look for the image of the Deity or presiding Spirit between the altar-groups of convoluted candelabra. And I see—only a mirror, a round, pale disk of polished metal, and my own face therein . . . Only a mirror! Symbolizing what?" Hearn has reached what he believes to be the heart of Japanese spirituality, hoping to see the face of the kami, or at least a portrayal of one. Instead, he finds nothing save a reflection of himself. He is smart enough to realize that it means something—but what? He would spend the rest of his life, during which he wrote more than a dozen books on Japanese spirituality and folklore, trying to decipher the riddle.

In Hearn's story I am reminded of my own attempts to talk to the invisible as a little girl, my own encounters with a spirituality only vaguely understood, the journey my own questions set me on. What was to me an altar was to my mother a shoebox. The shrine in the park where I had my epiphany was the same shrine I'd walked by countless times without thinking twice about it. What we find at shrines, makeshift, man-made, or natural, in the hills over Yokohama or anywhere else in the world, is what we bring to them.

For most of my life I, like many Japanese, only ever set out purposefully to visit a shrine once a year. It was "hatsumodé," literally "first visit," the year's very first prayer, traditionally performed after the stroke of midnight on New Year's Day. My parents started taking me to hatsumodé as soon as I was old enough to stay up late. When my younger sister reached an appropriate age, she joined us as well.

The itinerary was always the same: a simple supper of soba noodles, followed by a few hours of the nation's most popular year-end entertainment—the celebrity singing contest *Kohaku Uta Gassen* (*The Red and White Song Battle*), where Japan's top stars competed onstage for audience votes. It felt like all of Japan tuned in to this televised mic battle every year, and my parents inevitably timed our departure for a few minutes before the show ended, to beat the crowds.

It was a ten-minute walk from our house to the shrine.

Normally, the streets would be deserted at this hour, but hatsumodé meant many other families were out, making the same little pilgrimage we were. As we queued before the main altar for our turn to pay our respects, we'd sip umami-sweet amazaké, the nonalcoholic sediment from making rice wine, a traditional winter treat served up from a steaming cauldron to help ward off the chill. More than the prayer ritual itself—over in a moment, two quick bows, two claps, and a final bow—what I remember was the trip itself. Particularly as we grew older, hatsumodé represented a rare moment when we were all together, quietly walking and talking and just being a family in those first moments of a new year. The same scene played out at shrines across Japan, whether in the countryside, the suburbs, or the heart of the city.

"If you ask me, there's nothing better than ringing in the New Year in downtown Tokyo," wrote Haruki Murakami around this very same time, in 1982. "Every New Year's Eve, I eat soba noodles in Roppongi, then make my way to Shinjuku for a drink before catching a movie in Kabukicho. Then I head to Harajuku to read my fortune at Togo Shrine, stop for a cup of coffee, browse for some tunes at a record shop holding an all-night sale, have some tako-yaki from a street vendor, and finally return home to my neighborhood of Sendagaya, where I have a cup of consecrated saké at Hato-no-mori Shrine before turning in."

Not everyone celebrates hatsumodé with such Murakami-esque panache, of course, but huge numbers of Japanese do so in their own ways. In the three days after New Year's Day 2019, 100 million Japanese made hatsumodé visits to shrines and temples, big and small, all over Japan. A hundred million out of a population of what was then 126 million.

In survey after survey, anywhere from five to seven out

of ten Japanese claim not to have any religious beliefs at all—that religion plays no role in their day-to-day lives. Hatsumodé seems to suggest otherwise. But what draws us in? Simple inertia, the pull of tradition, plays a part. But there's another reason. Shrines are holy ground, but they are not somber, sectarian, or sepulchral; they are places to mingle with friends and neighbors, to celebrate, to live—to have *fun*, a word I can't recall hearing very often in my encounters with religion abroad. We come in hopes of contact with something beyond our day-to-day existences; on festival days and holidays, we do it through excitement and camaraderie, and in the usual everydays, we do it quietly, to restore and to heal. The grounds of Meiji Jingu are covered by acres of forest, an oasis of natural beauty curated within Tokyo's cyberpunk steel and concrete, a quiet reminder of where our spirituality first began: a womb of soil and stone, wood and water.

But in the end, even the grandest shrine is only a receptacle for what we bring to it. The point is to disengage from the static of the here and now and refocus on what we can't see or hear or touch but always feel, if we open our hearts. Just as the ancients did with their iwakura rock-seats, just as the modern-day masses jostle for hatsumodé. Just as a little girl once kneeled in front of a makeshift altar crafted from a shoebox.

I was only six back then, but I was already using spiritual tools as a way to fill a hole in my heart. I don't think I was precocious or special—I was simply tapping into something innately human, for in times of need, we all want to make contact with someone bigger than ourselves, who might have answers we don't.

I didn't know anything about Shinto as a little girl, but there were echoes of it in what I was doing. Years later, when

I began studying Shinto in earnest, I realized that shrines and altars are tools to remind us of the spiritual side to life, a safe haven of sorts that quietly coexists alongside our humdrum realities. Shrines are pretty much empty spaces; iwakura are just rocks; my shoebox was just a shoebox. But these things all served a similar purpose: to put a "pause" on your life for just a moment, the better to observe your own feelings and thoughts. They offer the opportunity for a little ritual in our lives, without any quid pro quo or expectation other than courteousness. This is why so many of my people, I suspect, don't see the act of praying at a shrine or a temple as a religious act—because they welcome all comers, making a visit feel refreshing rather than obligatory. Because they give us a little breathing room in the midst of a hectic day.

It isn't necessary to study the foundational stories of Shinto to incorporate this kind of thinking into one's life. I suspect few average Japanese know the tales in any but the broadest strokes. Even if one hasn't read the legends, the term *kami-sama* is an all-around, even almighty sort of honorific, so it can refer to any of the eight million kami individually or collectively.

There's nothing wrong with this at all. In fact, it's altogether common. But I wanted to know more. I think my fascination with the details of the individual kami mirrored other hungers within me. The photos of my mother hinted at complexities and subtleties lying beyond the day-to-day relationship I'd had with her, and the diaries of my great-grandfather hinted at a web of relationships I hadn't ever really considered before. I was starting to have questions. And questions are the start of journeys.

My studies of Shinto lore and visits to Shinto sites opened my eyes to new ways of thinking about my own culture and the world at large. This was empowering, but I knew my work was only beginning. Shinto is a powerful force in our culture, but it is by no means the only spiritual influence. In practice it is intertwined with another system imported from abroad: Buddhism.

Unlike Shinto, Buddhism does have holy texts, and sutras, and many different sects and schools. Over the many centuries since its arrival, Buddhism has had a profound effect on Japanese society, from art and architecture to culture and even politics. Buddhism as a religion is far better known abroad than is Shinto as a spirituality. So are its peculiarly Japanese manifestations, such as Zen, which in my experience is often used interchangeably with Buddhism as a whole, among non-Japanese laypeople. Perhaps because of this familiarity, there have been times when Japan has been called a Buddhist nation. In a certain sense, this isn't wrong—but neither, as I was about to learn, is it right.

CHAPTER 2

The Harmony of Conflict: Buddhism

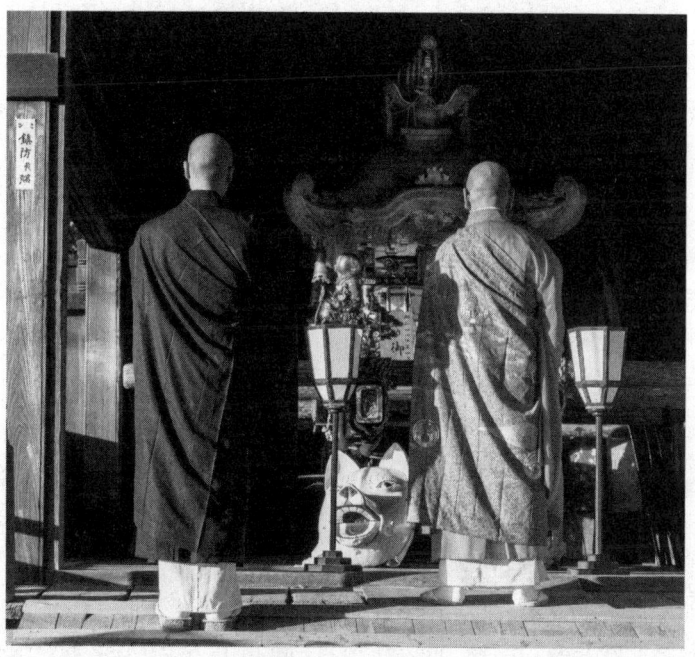

*Buddhist monks blessing a Shinto mikoshi float
at Myogonji temple in Aichi.*

If we want to see the degree to which Buddhism has entered into the history and life of the Japanese people, let us imagine that all the temples and the treasuries sheltered therein were completely destroyed. Then we should feel what a desolate place Japan would be in spite of all her natural beauty and kindly disposed people. The country would then look like a deserted house with no furniture, no pictures, no screens, no sculptures, no tapestries, no gardens, no flower arrangements, no Noh plays, no art of tea, and so on.

—D. T. Suzuki, *Zen and Japanese Culture*, 1959

Shinto isn't the only spiritual tradition in Japan, of course. It is joined by many other beliefs. But its oldest companion is Buddhism. Note I didn't say "rival." The deities of Shinto are known as kami. Those of Buddhism, hotoke. That's the official distinction, anyway. In colloquial speech, people are just as likely to use *kami* to refer to either or both.

Today the kami and hotoke coexist harmoniously at shrines and temples throughout Japan. But that harmony was hard-won, the product of a holy war fought over a millennium ago. The effects of that conflict can still be felt today. One of the biggest is that Shinto and Buddhist traditions have been so thoroughly integrated that it can often be hard to tell kami and hotoke apart. And as a result, it can be hard for many of us to explain if we are Shinto or Buddhist.

The idea that a person must identify with one or the other is not something that comes naturally to Japanese people. Traditionally, Shinto and Buddhism do not proselytize or strive for converts. To be honest, I don't even know what "convert" would mean in this context. I've never heard of a conversion ceremony, like the baptisms of Christian faith—you simply do things in one tradition or another, or don't. Even broad terms like *Shinto* or *Buddhism* fail to serve as boundaries. My Shinto Cultural Examinations textbook made that abundantly clear, explaining that there are kami out there being venerated in Shinto shrines that are clearly influenced by Buddhism, Taoism, and other foreign religions. Really, you could say the same about Japanese society as a whole. Professor D. T. Suzuki, who transmitted Zen philosophy to American tastemakers in the fifties, called Buddhism in Japan "an influence so pervasive, indeed, that those who are living in its midst are not at all conscious of it."

As I've said, I don't consider myself a religious person. And Buddhism is most definitely a religion with a capital *R*, an organized one, with believers all over the world. I have no background in Buddhist worship or studies. Yet I needed to grapple with the impact of Buddhist thinking on my society to understand myself. I studied Shinto through the cultural examinations, but Buddhism? I didn't have a clue as to how to approach it. There isn't any equivalent of those exams for Buddhism, because there are 156 sects and schools of faith registered in Japan. Which to pick? I had no idea. And, besides, choosing any given school wouldn't give me the big picture I was looking for. Because I wasn't interested in religion per se. I was interested in how faith can become culture, transforming from divine writ for believers into spiritual traditions for everyone—where it is practiced with neither belief nor disbelief but a sort of instinctive balance between the two.

How could I have this religious influence coursing through me, through my cultural DNA, without being conscious of it? Can one be *culturally* religious without being religiously religious? What does that even mean?

Resolving that question would take me to a great many places across many years and through many cultures. And it would end with a boat—a boat carrying gods from around the world, sailing merrily under the same flag, their enduring popularity in my country proof positive that harmony equals happiness. But not the kind of harmony you might think.

It all began with a meeting, back when I was still in high school. The occasion was my enrolling in an international exchange program run by an organization named Youth for Understanding.

There was an orientation. The organizers handed out sheets of paper titled "Useful Information for Your Stay in America." It described various dos and don'ts: "Don't take off your shoes when entering a home unless asked" and "Don't bow when you meet someone; just say 'hi'" and "Don't reflexively apologize; say 'excuse me' instead."

Another section covered "common questions Americans may ask," with a list of suggested responses. There were many, but today I remember only one: "What religion are the Japanese?" The suggested response was "I am a Buddhist."

Buddhist? I clearly remember the wave of puzzlement that washed over the attendees, including myself. One quizzical parent raised a hand and asked for clarification. The orientation leader replied, "I know it isn't necessarily the *right* answer, but it's the easiest, and least problematic. America is a religious country. We need to give them some kind of response."

This suggestion did more than confuse. It made me downright uncomfortable. I'd always pay my respects when

I went to one of our many Buddhist temples, dropping a coin in the collection box and praying at the main altar. But I'd never seen those visits as specifically religious acts. Did putting up Christmas decorations make me a Christian? I didn't think so. I also prayed at Shinto shrines from time to time, like everyone else I knew. So the more I thought about it, the less confident I felt declaring I was Buddhist to anyone. This wasn't out of any aversion to Buddhism. I just feared getting asked anything about it, for I wouldn't have had a clue about how to answer.

The exchange program placed me in a small Midwestern town about an hour and a half east of Indianapolis. A few days earlier I'd been living in Tokyo. Now "downtown" consisted of a post office, a gas station, a church, and a general store. Adjusting to life in a foreign country is daunting for anyone, but being dropped into the middle of rural America was even more of a shock for a big-city girl. I was a stranger in a strange land whose locals knew next to nothing about my home. I recall the proud owner of a new CD player pointedly asking if my country had anything like this marvelous new technology. It was a Sony, but I decided not to press the point.

I took a similar tack when Americans asked me about religion, dodging the question as best I could. Which was actually quite easy, given the fragmentary state of my conversational English at the time. This reticence, compounded by my inability to convey anything coherent about Japanese spirituality in the first place, led my host mother to conclude that I didn't believe in God at all.

She was a devout Christian who went to church twice every Sunday, in the morning for the sermon and the late afternoon for Bible study, and the idea of having a (perceived) atheist under her roof was anathema. She decided I would accompany the family to services every week.

Much of the content at church, whether sermons or Bible excerpts, sailed right over my head. To everyone's credit there, I was never forced or even urged, really, to formally adopt Christianity. But there wasn't any question that I would be there, that I somehow *needed* to be there. Perhaps my host mother assumed some of her religion would rub off on me, eventually. Out of boredom, I began approaching these weekly visits as a form of cultural studies, in the manner of an anthropologist absorbing the ways of some far-flung tribe. It was the first time I'd seen a preacher preach, heard a congregation rise in song, sung along to hymns like "Jesus Loves Me," and taken communion wafers.

I was even pressed into service for the annual nativity scene. I'd heard the story of Jesus's birth even before coming to America, but I never imagined I'd be playing a part in an actual re-creation. Ours was held in a makeshift manger arranged on a parishioner's lawn, complete with live goats borrowed from a neighboring farm. My host sister played Mary, cradling a baby-doll Jesus; for some reason, I was enlisted to play Joseph. It struck me as odd for a young Asian woman to be asked to play the part of a hirsute older man, but I appreciated the spirit of inclusiveness and gave it my best shot. Outfitted with a robe, headscarf, and scratchy dime-store costume beard, I took my assigned spot in the lineup. The organizers provided a small space heater, but it was on the other side of the manger, and as time went on, I could feel the heat sapping from my bones. I stood patiently for an hour, shepherd's crook quivering in trembling hand, as members of the congregation gathered to view our little tableaux. I was struck by their reverence, their murmurs of appreciation, how genuinely touching they seemed to find the scene. But the thing that stuck with me most of all, besides the memory of that itchy beard, is just how frigid a December night in Indiana could be.

....

SUPERFICIALLY, AT LEAST, IT MAKES A CERTAIN SENSE THAT my orientation leaders would advise us to claim we were Buddhist. Many, if not most, Japanese homes contain Buddhist altars. As anyone who has visited Japan knows, Buddhist temples are a common sight—the more famous ones are literal tourist attractions. You might even catch sight of a monk chanting sutras for alms in front of a train station. Buddhist art represents some of our most precious artistic heritage, while Buddhist statuary, particularly the little bodhisattvas known as jizo, can be found along roads and trails practically everywhere. And when we finally shuffle off this mortal coil, Buddhist funerals are the norm.

Shinto, on the other hand? No scriptures. No evangelists. No statuary. The kami may be everywhere in their infinite multitude, but their forms are invisible, even unknowable. The only conspicuous manifestations of Shinto belief are iwakura and shrines, with their hempen ropes and paper streamers and tori'i gates. What do they mean? *Saa,* the average Japanese might say—*I wonder.* Or maybe: *Oh, that's just Shinto.* Neither of which is going to satisfy the truly curious, particularly those raised in traditions of evangelistic religions.

And there's an even bigger reason why one might portray Japan as a Buddhist country. One of our nation's founding fathers, so to speak, was a Buddhist by the name of Shotoku Taishi—the Prince of Holy Virtue. We know his story from *Chronicles of Japan,* which was written in 712 CE. While it is difficult to determine fact from fiction in such an ancient document, there is no question that the period in which he is said to have lived is precisely when the spiritualities of Japan and the outside world began to mix. It describes a conflict that erupted between supporters of native beliefs, so intertwined in daily life that nobody had even thought to name them, and proponents of Buddhism, a flashy and seductive interloper from across the seas.

Every Japanese person knows Shotoku, because we're taught about him starting in grade school. And depictions of him graced our paper currencies for much of the twentieth century, making his beatific countenance a part of daily life. He stands astride the crossroads of history and legend, something akin to America's George Washington, with as many or even more myths surrounding him. He's often portrayed as a sort of spiritual superman. He was capable of holding lucid conversations from the moment he was born, they say, and as an adult capable of conversing with ten people simultaneously. He had a horse that could fly, the legends go, and one day landed atop Mount Fuji—making him the first to summit that sacred peak. The list goes on.

Back in 574 CE, when Shotoku is said to have been born, Japan was a diplomatic backwater ruled by the whims of long-feuding warlord clans. By the time he died in 622 CE, he had established the beginnings of a centralized government, putting his nation on the regional map as a cultural force. He was a prince who would never become emperor, due to the byzantine feudal politics of the era, but he exerted a great influence over Japan's leadership from behind the scenes as a regent, the adviser to the throne.

Already by Shotoku's birth, Buddhists and believers of domestic religious traditions were clashing. A big part of Buddhism's appeal was its grand presence and physicality, so different from that of familiar old native beliefs. Even the kami adept who tended shrines didn't claim to know what the kami actually looked like. The kami could be *sensed* in the rising sun or an awesome clap of thunder, felt in the majesty of the waterfall or mountain, but they couldn't be *seen*. Buddhist statuary portrayed its deities in glorious three dimensions, with evocative expressions and dynamic poses. The statuary and sutras, and the highly trained monks who tended them in magnificently ornamented temples, hinted at profound truths beyond the shores of Japan. And unlike Shinto, which tended to focus on the earthly realm, Buddhism provided detailed road maps for the afterlife, the myriad paths of which converged in a mind-bendingly beautiful Pure Land. It all combined to make Buddhism both a religion and something more. It was cutting-edge, aspirational— even stylish.

Fifty years of hostilities between the believers of Buddhism and believers of domestic faiths culminated in a great battle. Shotoku fought on the side of the Buddhists, and their decisive victory that day gave him free rein to promote Buddhism throughout the land. One of his first acts after taking power as regent was to author a document called the Seventeen-Article Constitution. Unlike a modern-day constitution, it did not elaborate laws and rights but rather outlined morals and virtues. Key to it all was the concept of wa—harmony. The very first article reads that "wa wo motte totoshi tonasu"—"harmony should be cherished and quarrels avoided." The second article states that people should respect what he called the "three treasures": the Buddha himself, the teachings of Buddha, and Buddhist priests. Only in article three does the constitution mention the authority of the imperial line.

Shotoku is famed as a fighter for Buddhism, but his enshrining of wa as the nation's top virtue might rank as his most enduring legacy. Wa was in fact the name by which Japan was once known, long, long ago: Yamato, written with the characters "great" and "wa." Wa is so profoundly intertwined with our image that it is a synonym for things Japanese: *washi* meaning "Japanese paper," or *washoku* meaning "Japanese food," to name only two of countless examples. The concept of wa is woven so deeply into the fabric of Japanese culture that it might even be called the fabric of Japanese culture itself.

Like the word *kami*, the meaning of *wa* can be difficult to convey. It does mean harmony, and it also encompasses nuances of tranquility, gentleness, amicability, and acceptance. Yet there is a dark side to it as well. Like many powerful ideas, wa has been warped by those so inclined, as seen in a trite Japanese homily: "The nail that sticks up is hammered down." This doesn't mean consensus. It means obedience, conformity, prioritizing the group over the individual, crushing difference to *simulate* consensus.

But true harmony can never be achieved through brute force. Real wa isn't about uniformity at all. In fact, it is precisely the opposite: an acknowledgment and embrace of opposing ideas, a search for some sort of balance or middle ground between them, taking the best of each with the aim of achieving something bigger than either on its own. Savvy people knew this. The celebrated surrealist pop artist Taro Okamoto believed that "true harmony only emerges from conflict," and Soichiro Honda, founder of the famed automotive company, declared "disharmony the building block of harmony."

Shotoku's face actually adorned the 10,000-yen bill for almost three decades, from 1958 until 1986. Perhaps fittingly, he was finally retired at a particularly unharmonious time for my country. In 1986 the Japanese economy was booming, to the point that foreign pundits (and more than a few Japanese people) thought we were going to take over the world. In one sense, it's hard to blame them. It was the kind of time when businessmen ruled the roost, when tycoons bought up foreign sports teams, golf courses, landmarks, and priceless art, and average folks became paper millionaires simply from owning a little real estate. Our government jousted endlessly with Western leaders over trade deficits and the disruption of local markets by cheaper Japanese products. Today we call it the Bubble era.

My exchange program to America coincided with the Bubble's peak in 1989. It didn't take long for me to notice that Americans saw Japanese businessmen as something akin to enemies of the state. I still remember going to see the movie *Back to the Future Part II*, where a heavily accented "Mr. Fujitsu" mercilessly fires the hopeless, grown-up Marty McFly. I'd loved the first *Back to the Future*, which had been a big hit in Japan, too, but this scene made me cringe. I know the joke was only a reflection of an era, but Japanese businessmen weren't monsters to me. My own father was a businessman. So were the fathers of most of my friends. They certainly didn't seem like the venal Asian antagonists I kept seeing in American movies and on TV, an interchangeable army of samurai salarymen marching in lockstep, intent on poaching American jobs.

That said, there was a kernel of truth in these overly reductive portrayals. The group ruled, in the Japan of the day. A famous Red Bull–like energy drink called Regain ran television commercials exhorting Japanese businessmen to "fight 24 hours a day." To strive for success seems like a wonderful ambition, and it is, on a personal level. But this wasn't about individuals. You were expected to sublimate your own dreams and desires for the good of the organization—whether it be family, school, or company—for the conventional wisdom went that they would take care of you in turn. But this left no room for any kind of deviation from the norm, or personal expression that rocked the boat.

This thinking even extended to sports. "The concept and practice of group harmony or *wa* is what most dramatically differentiates Japanese baseball from the American game," wrote Robert Whiting in a 1989 bestseller titled *You Gotta Have Wa*. It chronicled the struggles of all-American major leaguers who were lured to play in Japan with eye-popping Bubble-era salaries, then were punished if they ever dared outshine their new teammates. (Whiting called *the nail that sticks up is hammered down* "practically the national slogan.")

Again, it was my trip to America that opened my eyes to a question I hadn't even thought to ask: Was Japan valuing harmony, or was it valuing something else? I never really questioned my nation's obsession with group consensus and social harmony until I went to America. In fact, our being told to claim Buddhist beliefs was a sort of wa, in that our minders didn't want us to "stick up" in a Christian-majority country that might "hammer us down." I was only a teenager, and took it for granted that I was but a bit player in bigger, more important associations of family, school, and society. Last names always come first in Japan; if someone asked who I was, I'd answer with my family name and the school I went to. Such was my face to the public world. And within this cultural cocoon, I never thought of myself as Japanese, for like those of native faiths before the arrival of Buddhism, I didn't have anyone non-Japanese to whom I might compare myself. But that was all about to change. I was going to a country where personal names came first.

The public school that Youth for Understanding placed

me at in Indiana was small, with the kindergarten, elementary school, junior high school, and high school all housed in the same compound. I vividly remember my first day of school. I was incredibly nervous, of course. In Tokyo, I navigated to school aboard a series of trains that crisscrossed an urban landscape. Here I boarded a giant yellow school bus with green vinyl seats that carried us over a series of country roads. And once we got to school, I felt the eyes of students and faculty alike, all focused on me, the first Japanese person many of them had ever seen. I went to greet the principal in his office. Then my very first school day in America began.

The first thing that struck me was how different each student looked. Different skin tones and eye colors, different hair colors and styles. I went to an all-girls high school in Japan. All of us looked pretty much the same, with similar skin tones and straight, jet-black hair, for the school regulated our hair colors and even styles. We wore uniforms. No exotic hairstyles were allowed. Jewelry and even makeup were strictly forbidden. The Americans sported earrings, boys and girls both. Girls wore makeup and permed their hair, then fluffed it to the heavens with dryers and extra-hold hair spray. Everyone wore different clothes. The halls were a riot of color, of jeans and miniskirts, sneakers and even high heels.

Everybody welcomed me warmly as their first exchange student from Asia. I was asked all sorts of questions about my home country. "What kind of food do Japanese people eat?" "Do they celebrate Thanksgiving in Japan?" "Do you all drive to school, too?" I did my best to answer in my limited English. My favorite was from a kindergartner who asked me if there was air in Japan. She reminded me of myself at her age. When I was little, I thought there was a planet called America, and I dreamed of getting big enough to ride a rocket to it someday.

In a sense I had been right, for America did feel like another planet in a lot of ways, some obvious, like the clothing, others less so. One of the biggest things that took getting used to was that Americans preferred specific answers to the more open-ended responses common in Japan. In Japan, where nobody wanted to rock the boat with replies that might upset the listener, speakers often spoke indirectly, while listeners were expected to "read the air"—what in English you'd call "reading between the lines," intuiting what the speaker meant through subtle contextual cues.

The stereotypical example is Japan's unwillingness to say a direct "no." In Japanese, if one is asked to do something that isn't possible, the usual response is "muzukashii desu ne"—"I think that'd be difficult." A native speaker would immediately recognize this as a flat-out refusal. In the States, however, a listener would be moved to probe deeper. Why is it difficult? What might be done to make it easier? This would in turn ruffle the Japanese, who saw "that's difficult" as an idiom meaning "no way." *Why won't this person meet me halfway?* thinks the aggravated American. *Why won't this person stop hounding me?* thinks the aggravated Japanese.

Over the course of the year, I had to retrain myself to be more specific in my speaking, no matter how minor the subject may have seemed. If I were asked if I liked apples, for instance, and answered "yes," a flurry of return serves would follow: *What kind? McIntosh or Golden Delicious? How do you like to eat them? As is or in a pie?* On the other hand, answering "no" to virtually anything demanded a detailed justification of why. This was particularly hard for me, as in Japan, listeners tended not to probe too deeply into the negative, lest the speaker be cornered into talking about something they'd rather not. Reading the air was seen as a social grace.

Most challenging of all, however, was when I was faced with questions that didn't have clear-cut answers. These would inevitably lead me to be asked my own opinions on the topic. *How do you feel about that, Hiroko?* or *What would you do in that situation?* This was something that, quite frankly, didn't happen in Japan, particularly Japan of that era. We "nails" were expected to stay hammered firmly down. An opinion equated to sticking up. But I quickly discovered that in America, a nail that stays down gets ignored. If I failed to assert myself, I'd end up unnoticed, a wallflower, watching the world go by. Peer pressure was a huge boon in this regard. I needed to act more assertively in order to keep up with my friends. So I did.

By the end of that year, I'd come to a realization. Harmony doesn't have to equal uniformity. It doesn't have to mean obedience, or staying quiet when you have something to say. There are lots of different people out there, and lots of different ideas.

Several years after I finished the exchange program, I went back to the US for undergraduate and graduate programs. In those classrooms, debate was encouraged and rewarded. Here I learned how to construct arguments to make my points in papers and discussions, to express my opinions in ways I'd never even considered in the Japanese educational system. But I saw downsides to this approach, too. Discussions sometimes felt like arenas, where the knives were out for any sign of weakness, and everyone was a critic. The loudest voices inevitably dominated the conversation, regardless of the quality of points they were making. And stickier topics could quickly devolve into invective and insult.

I learned a great many things from my experiences in the American educational system, but I wasn't exactly converted by them. I still toggle between Japanese and American forms of expression today. And that's fine, because harmony—real harmony—isn't just a goal but is also a process. Harmony is dynamic and ever-changing because people are dynamic and ever-changing. Harmony is hard, but it's worth it, because it makes us better and stronger—all of us. I had always brushed off the story of Shotoku being able to understand ten people talking at him simultaneously as a flight of historical fantasy, but when you think about it, maybe that isn't such a bad symbol of harmony after all. Listening to different voices, then weaving them into something new, all while letting each shine in its own way.

It might seem Shotoku's Seventeen-Article Constitution represented a total victory for Buddhism in Japan. Yet this was never, even at the peak of hostilities, a holy war in the sense we think of today. The advocates for Buddhism certainly wanted to crush their rivals. But theirs was a struggle over power, not theology. Erasing local beliefs was never part of the plan. Buddhism was, at this point in history, exclusively for the chosen few, the rulers and aristocrats. Shotoku viewed its adoption as much through the lenses of politics and diplomacy as through the lens of religion.

Paradoxically, Buddhism's triumph allowed the kami to endure. Defeat forced kami worshippers to grapple with the idea of coexistence. Until the arrival of Buddhism, there wasn't any need to think about this sort of thing, because there wasn't anything to which native beliefs might be compared. The phrase "Kannagara no michi," literally "The Way of Kami," would not enter the Japanese lexicon for another thirty or so years after Shotoku's time, when it was used to describe Japan's blend of religious beliefs in *Chronicles of Ja-*

pan: "The Emperor embraces Buddhism and respects the Way of Kami." Even then, a millennium ago, we were patching the quilt of beliefs that endures today.

We call this "shinbutsu shugo"—"the merging of kami and bodhisattvas." In essence, we live in a remix culture for spirituality. When something new comes along, we tend to incorporate rather than replace. As a result, there has never been one god here. With "yaoyorozu-no-kami"—"eight million kami," there's always room for more deities—or new interpretations of old ones. Having spent time in places where the conflicts between religious beliefs seem intractable, such as Jerusalem and the West Bank, or within the US in recent years, I think about my nation's spiritual harmony a lot. They hint that coexistence isn't a pipe dream. The evidence is all around us—not only at holy sites like shrines and temples but also inside our homes.

TODAY, MY MORNINGS INEVITABLY FOLLOW THE SAME PATtern. After going through my morning ablutions, I head downstairs to my office, where I place a small cup of water atop the bookshelf. That spot, the highest in the room, is where I have my kamidana—literally, an "altar for the kami."

I started feeling the need for one about five or six years back, as I began accumulating talismans from shrines and other religious objects during my studies. It just didn't feel right to pile them up in a corner or something, so I made a space for them atop the bookshelf. Over time I added to it and found myself attending to it every morning. It became a kamidana.

Now I can't imagine living without one. No matter how busy I am, no matter how early I have to leave in the morning, I always make time to change the water and say a quiet prayer of thanks to the kami I've invited into my home. It isn't anything fancy. I don't really even put it into words. It's more a feeling: *Thanks for giving me another day.* I don't mean it as though I'm sick or anything. But it's a fact that life is short. Every day we get is another opportunity to do, to change, to be.

I never had a kamidana in my house growing up. My parents had only the more popular butsudan, a household Buddhist altar, which is commonly used to display the memorial tablets of deceased relatives. In this we were not alone; kamidana ownership has long been on the decline in Japan. In a 2019 survey, less than 40 percent of respondents claimed to own one, and of those, only a little over 20 percent said they interacted with them on a regular basis.

Still, it isn't uncommon for a home to have one, and there are indications that their use is growing once again. Marie Kondo has spoken of kamidana in her books and also of the one she keeps in her home. In a 2018 interview, she elaborated on its role in her daily routine: "After waking up, I open all of the windows, let the breeze in, and then burn incense. We have a Japanese-style *kamidana*. On the shelf, there is some salt, some rice, and some evergreen fronds, and I'll give this a once-over, freshening things up. Then I'll pray for the health of my family and friends."

She continues, "This is not a religious thing, really, at all. It's just for me to take this time every morning to feel gratitude."

Haruki Murakami has written about kamidana as well. In the afterword to the Japanese edition of *The Great Gatsby*, the translation of which had been a lifelong ambition of his, he wrote: "Metaphorically speaking, I had placed *Gatsby* securely on my kamidana, the high shelf that serves as a shrine to the Shinto gods, and lived my life glancing up at it from time to time."

Linguistically speaking, an altar is a place where religious rites are performed, while a shrine is a place where something holy is honored. A kamidana combines aspects of both. They can be simple boxlike arrangements, or gorgeously elaborate structures that resemble Shinto shrines in miniature, complete with details like little balconies and staircases. Smaller ones are designed to be set atop a shelf; the largest models need to be mounted on a wall, like cabinetry. They are almost always made of wood, traditionally fragrant cedar.

Whether simple or grand, a new kamidana is nothing more than a box until it is activated by placing one or more ofuda talismans inside. Ofuda are consecrated wooden tablets or slips of Japanese paper. They're sold at Shinto shrines, avatars of the kami being worshipped there. Once you have chosen a talisman to bring home, the most important thing is your taking care of the kamidana—your showing of gratitude to the kami that you've asked inside. Praying to a kami at a shrine versus a kamidana is kind of like the difference between polite acquaintance and being on first-name terms. I don't mean that one is better than the other—this isn't a competition. But inviting a kami into your home implies aspiring to a certain degree of intimacy. And that's what a kamidana is all about.

In Japan, it isn't hard to find premade kamidana. They're sold at shops specializing in religious paraphernalia, and any department store worth its salt will have a selection as well. This might come as a surprise given the drop in ownership over the years, but as with so many other things, COVID-19 upended that trend, too. Trapped indoors by lockdowns, with group festivities like hatsumodé canceled, sales of kamidana soared over the course of 2019 and 2020. When faced with trying times, many Japanese returned to the kami, and the comfort of ritual, to help them through.

Traditionally we reach out to the kami in our kamidana through offerings of water and salt, refreshed daily, and sprigs of sakaki evergreens, changed every few weeks. But there are no hard-and-fast rules beyond the showing of gratitude, which means in practice the rituals are often as distinctive as their owners.

Kondo's use of incense is interesting, as it isn't really associated with Shinto. But it is an integral part of Buddhist rituals—lighting a stick is a common practice at temples, and dropping powdered incense into a censer a key part of Buddhist funeral ceremonies. Kondo's routine is yet another example of the facility with which Japanese switch between symbols and rituals as needed, often without even realizing it.

Active kamidana take on the characteristics of their keepers, and mine is no different. Perhaps because I visit shrines so regularly, I didn't feel the need to purchase a fancy construction for my home. Instead, I arranged my kamidana myself—a collection of objects I gathered to watch over the room. Like Kondo's, it incorporates a mixture of Shinto and Buddhist elements: a gathering of favorite kami and deities. When I refresh the little cup of water placed before them every morning, it is in the same spirit as greeting a family member with a steaming cup of coffee.

Perhaps the single most precious object atop my altar is a carving of Daikokuten, a deity of fortune and wealth. It's more than a hundred years old, and showing its age. Roughly the size of a softball, it was coated in some sort of pitch-like substance to protect it from the elements. Over the decades the coating dulled to a sooty black, shrunk and cracked, revealing the naked wood beneath in patches, pockmarked here and there with dozens of wormholes from tiny residents long since disappeared.

I found him at a small antique store in Kamakura, a popular tourist destination an hour away from Tokyo on the Shonan seaside. It was run by an old lady who hadn't bothered giving her little boutique a name, or even hanging a sign out front. In fact, its frosted-glass windows hid the contents of the store so thoroughly that many passersby undoubtedly mistook it for a private residence. But the door was open a crack when I walked by, and I'd caught sight of the interior. It stopped me in my tracks, as though I'd been beckoned.

The space couldn't have been more than twelve feet on a side, a small square room crammed to the rafters with ephemera, more like a storehouse than a store. The scent of dust, of wood, of cloth, of age was in the air. Shelves groaned with ceramics, archaic tools, baskets of vintage hairpins, incense burners, dolls, statues, and more. There was even an old mino—a straw raincoat of the sort worn by travelers in the premodern era—tacked to a wall. There was barely any room to maneuver inside; two customers would need to pass each other cheek to jowl. Yet it didn't feel claustrophobic. It was actually quite cozy, being surrounded by all these old mementos. You could sense that each and every one had been picked by the owner, that each had a story. So many antique shops I've been to feel like de facto dumping grounds. Not so this one. Everything in there had its own little aura.

Among her wares were a number of Buddhist statues, as varied as the contents of the shop itself. One was gilt. Another was carved wood. One was tall. Another rotund. Some looked new, while others showed their age, their wear a résumé of previous lives worshipped by someone, some-where, before winding up here on a shelf in a store without a name by the seaside.

For some reason, one of the statues caught my eye: the roly-poly, sooty black Daikokuten.

"It's more than a hundred years old," said the proprie-tress, noticing my interest.

"May I take a closer look?" I asked.

"Certainly."

It was much lighter than I expected. Normally, Daiko-kuten carries a mallet, a swing of which is said to bring good fortune. But this statue didn't have one. The entire right hand was cracked clean off. A true collector would have seen this as a detriment, I'm sure. But I wasn't inter-ested in Daikokuten as an investment. I just liked his smile.

"Antiques are 'travelers,'" I heard the old lady say from over my shoulder.

"Travelers?"

"Well, they travel from owner to owner," she explained. "Almost anything has the potential to become an antique, but some have more of a knack for traveling than others. Those that don't have the knack get thrown away and dis-appear."

I smiled when I heard this. I have a clay statue of a ta-nuki, a raccoon-dog trickster from folklore. It was made in the Meiji Era, at the turn of the twentieth century. It was intended to be displayed in a garden, outdoors, which is where I had initially placed mine. But not long after, a storm came, and I found myself instinctively bringing it inside. When my husband saw it sitting in a corner of the room, he laughed and said it had tricked me into keeping it indoors. I suspect it has pulled this trick on earlier owners, too, as it is in mint condition.

"When you think about it," she continued, "the owners of antiques don't really 'own' them. More like 'borrowing' them. It's as though we were chosen by them, to spend a little time together before they resume their journey to the next destination, whenever the time comes."

I wanted Daikokuten to spend some time with me before heading off on his next journey. And so I paid the asking price and took him home. He's been watching over my house from the kamidana ever since.

This particular Daikokuten may have been "in transit" for more than a hundred years, but that's a blink of an eye in the history of Daikokuten himself. His origins can be traced back to Shiva, the famed Hindu destroyer of worlds. At times, Shiva was known as Mahakala, the "Great Black One," and this incarnation was adopted by Buddhists. In Japan, Mahakala was conflated with a Shinto kami called Okuninushi, as the first kanji characters in Okuninushi's name can also be pronounced "daikoku," a homonym for "great black." Thus transformed from fearsome destroyer Shiva to chubby and affable Daikokuten, he is famed throughout Japan not only as a bearer of good fortune but also as one of a group with the cheery name the Seven Gods of Happiness.

....

THE SEVEN GODS OF HAPPINESS—ALSO KNOWN IN TRANS-
lation as the Seven Lucky Gods—are a motley crew of deities from disparate religions. Multicultural, mixed gender, and religiously diverse, it's a particularly progressive group of gods. Of the seven, only one, Ebisu, a kami of business and the seas, has any indigenous Japanese background. The rest are imports from Buddhist, Hindu, and Taoist beliefs, remixed as incarnations of fertility, longevity, and other

good fortune. One of them, Hotei, is even based on a real person, a monk from long ago.

Today, portrayals of the seven are ubiquitous in Japanese society. They often appear in a ra takarabuné (treasure ship) riding the waves, smiling and partying together, a symbol of prosperity and joy for all with the good fortune to see them.

Just like Daikokuten, each has its own history. Many were and still are venerated on their own, as the patron saints of various professions. The rotund Ebisu and Daikokuten served the fortunes of merchants; Benzaiten, a beautiful female kami carrying a lute, served as avatar of the arts. Others served as avatars for the fortunes everyone might want: Fukurokuju and Jurojin, kami of longevity; Bishamonten, a kami of power and authority; the plump Hotei, an avatar of fertility and happiness.

It seems to have been the citizens of Kyoto who first "packaged" these disparate deities into an ad hoc spiritual team in the 1400s. The occasion was the end of yet another protracted civil war of the sort that broke out often in those days. Jubilant residents staged a procession to the Fushimi Inari Shrine, dressed in costumes of what would later become known as the Seven Gods of Happiness. (Fushimi Inari is still there today; you may have seen photos of its pathways, framed by rows of crimson tori'i gates.) This holy cosplay was a form of religious celebration, of course, but it was equally if not more so a kind of carnival, fueled by excitement at the bad times being behind, with good things in store ahead. We should all be so lucky.

Then as now, kami were everywhere. But kami were powerful and stern presences on high—that was why you took such care venerating them, lest ingratitude kindle their anger. The Seven Gods of Happiness represented a new face of kami. They loved to party and brought prosperity to those around them. They were expressive, exuberant, and downright fun. Who wouldn't want to hang out with them? The Seven Gods of Happiness were serious business—everyone wanted good fortune in their lives—but they injected a healthy dose of play into the prayers of Japanese.

The down-to-earth nature of the Seven Gods of Happiness made them the canvas for an ever-changing array of pop cultural fads and trends over the centuries to come. Put a picture of the seven under your pillow on New Year's Day, an old saying went, and you'd have a great first dream of the year. And pilgrimages to shrines and temples venerating the individual gods became a popular post–New Year's pastime: Take the time out of your busy life to greet each of the seven, and you'd be sure to boost your chances of fortune in the year to come.

Seven Gods of Happiness pilgrimages remain a popular New Year's tradition today. They're held in communities throughout Japan, and don't require any kind of religious commitment or connection to participate. I recently did one in the Tokyo neighborhood of Shitaya, which provides manga-style illustrated maps to the locations of each of its effigies of the Seven Gods. Participants purchase a special card decorated with their faces; the idea is that you make your way to the spot venerating each one, say a prayer of thanks, and get a stamp from the shrine or temple staff. It was a cold winter morning when I set out on the pilgrimage with my husband; we initially got lost but ran into a group of participants who were just finishing and helped us get back on track. Both that community spirit, and the experience itself, reinforced just how much the Seven Gods of

Happiness embody Japan's patchwork of spiritual traditions. We began at a Shinto shrine, but the course took us through a Shugendo temple, and we ended at a Buddhist temple.

And while this tradition may have roots in times of old, it has modern twists. One of the temples placed a capsule-toy vending machine out front. It was filled with miniature hollow ceramic figurines of Daikokuten that contained written fortunes inside. I couldn't resist, and spent three hundred yen, the equivalent of a few dollars, to get one of my own. Out popped a little Daikokuten with a cute smile, bearing a fortune carefully folded inside. I honestly don't even remember what it said, but it didn't matter, because I just wanted to take this happy little figurine home. Whatever fortunes the year might hold, I figured I'd be able to navigate them with this tiny Daikokuten on my desktop. He is sitting here as I type these words.

The experience reminded me of how, when I was young and my family would tromp off to the neighborhood shrine for hatsumodé, that first prayer of the New Year, we'd inevitably see a portrait of the Seven Gods of Happiness. It would be posted by the priest as part of the holiday decorations, showing them bobbing happily in their boat, carrying felicitations for a prosperous year to come. And whenever my dad saw the picture, he'd point a finger and inevitably recite the same anecdote.

Dad was an entrepreneur. His companies always dealt with cars: buying them, leasing them, servicing them. Automobiles were the lens through which he viewed life, particularly during Japan's boom times of the eighties. "Cars weren't invented in Japan," he'd tell me. "Americans created them. Japanese adopted them, because we saw their potential, and we improved them and made our country strong with them.

"It's just like the Seven Gods of Happiness. All of them are from different places, but we took them and put them in the same boat, and they're stronger for it. So are we. Differences are good things. If you can respect them, they can help make bigger, better things."

My father was an unusually forward-thinking man for his time. In an era when many Japanese still questioned the worth of sending women to four-year colleges, he gave his blessing to my traveling far and wide, from the comfortable suburban neighborhood where he raised us to the cornfields of the American Midwest and the deserts of the Middle East, from a junior college in Japan to postgraduate studies abroad.

After returning home and finishing high school, I went to a two-year college in Tokyo, took a full-time job at a big company in the city for a few years, and then went back to the US for a full university education. It was there, during those studies, that I learned the word *secular*, a word I found useful whenever people asked me about Japanese religion. "Oh, Japan is a secular country," I'd say, or "We Japanese are a secular people." We didn't go to temples or shrines with any of the regularity many Americans I knew went to church, so this simple answer worked. Thus, I was "secular."

Or so I thought, until I spent a summer in the Middle East.

Set on a beautiful hilltop surrounded by olive trees, the Tantur Ecumenical Institute was founded by the Vatican and run by the University of Notre Dame. I was there in the summer of 1995, as a research assistant to two of my professors. The institute also happened to be located right next to the border between Jerusalem and Bethlehem. From the building we could see the Israeli military checkpoint dividing Israel and the West Bank.

I was a political science major; religion wasn't on my agenda. But the city of Jerusalem had other plans in store. It is, of course, holy ground for Christians, Muslims, and Jews alike. This brought me into contact with a great many of the devout during my stay. Jews invited me for Shabbat on many Friday evenings. Muslims took me to see the Dome of the Rock. The Christians who ran the institute graciously provided me with meals every day, even letting me raid the kitchen's refrigerator if I was hungry after hours.

The more I spent time with these deeply religious people, the less confident I began to feel about describing Japan, or the Japanese, or even myself as "secular." I didn't consider myself Christian or Muslim or Jewish. I had no sense of worshipping a specific god in the way that they did. Yet still I found myself moved by their faiths, to the point where I felt I could even share their feelings of awe at spending daily life in the shadow of the divine. *I'm not Buddhist*, I found myself thinking. *But I'm not an atheist, either. So what am I?*

By process of elimination, I arrived at a singular solution: "I'm Japanese." This wasn't about religion but culture. At first I thought this was going back to square one, but I was wrong. It was the beginning of a new understanding. As I mentioned earlier, a majority of Japanese claim not to hold any religious beliefs at all. In 2024, the Pew Research Center surveyed the citizens of 102 nations about the importance of religion in their lives; my nation ranked dead last. Yet Japan is also home to some 84,000 Shinto shrines and 76,000 Buddhist temples. By way of comparison, we have "only" 55,000 convenience stores. Anyone who's spent any time in Japanese cities knows how ubiquitous a presence those stores are—and there are more than triple the number of shrines and temples out there. We "non-religious" Japanese spend our days surrounded by the divine, after all.

We are a nation of adopters and remixers, mixing and matching for our spiritual needs. It comes so naturally to us that I couldn't see it until I went abroad. There the seeds of understanding were planted: Not being able to explicitly define my beliefs wasn't a weakness at all. It was a strength.

The Seven Gods of Happiness are a perfect example. "A Buddhist, a Shinto, and a Taoist deity ride in a boat . . ." sounds like the beginning of a joke, but there's something very serious and important at play here. To an outsider, the seven must seem a symbol of interfaith tolerance, coming as they do from so many backgrounds, domestic and foreign, male and female. But you'd be hard-pressed to find a Japanese person who saw them that way. In fact, you'd have a hard time finding anyone who knew much of their history, or could reel off the names of all seven, beyond Ebisu and Daikokuten and Benzaiten, at the drop of a hat. The Seven Gods of Happiness may have come from different places, but today they're all Japanese kami to us, in the sense that they are all spiritual beings. They aren't merely tolerating each other; they're actually happy together.

They seem so comfortable, but I think they're really a symbol of *leaving* your comfort zone. We fear leaving our comfort zones because it raises the possibility of encountering unexpected things. It's a gamble, for some can delight, while others disturb or even outrage.

Leaving one's country for another is one of the biggest departures from a comfort zone of all—you're leaving behind the familiarity of your culture, and whether we admit it or not, our cultures are integral parts of our identities.

To put it in the context of the Seven Gods of Happiness, when you "sail" into unfamiliar waters, your "boat" will be rocked by "waves" of differences—ways of looking at spirituality, customs, manners, you name it. In turn, your differences reverberate and rock other boats. When you are a stranger in a strange land, it is very tempting to obfuscate or outright deny aspects of yourself to try and calm the waters.

I was told to call myself a Buddhist not because I was a Buddhist but to give me a rapid way of shutting down religious inquiries. I didn't exactly follow that suggestion, but I achieved the same result by avoiding the subject as much as I could. Once I learned the word *secular*, I quickly grasped its utility as a nondenominational way to deflect conversations on spiritual topics. I clung to it like a shield. Phrases like "my culture is secular" or "Japan is a secular society" formed an invisible wall around me, freeing me from having to get confrontational and say, "I'd rather not talk about it." Secular drew a line between me and the world.

Drawing lines is easy, because they're simple rejections. What's hard is rejecting rejection itself. Wrestling with the contradictions head-on, incorporating what works and leaving behind what doesn't, all the while still acknowledging the whole. It's tough to do this because engaging with someone honestly means making yourself vulnerable. That vulnerability makes it much easier for you to get hurt by others rejecting you. But in vulnerability can also be found the seeds of true growth. I didn't go to America to reject my own culture. Nor did I go because I wanted to embrace America's. What I wanted to do was to take some Americanness into my boat, so to speak, in hopes of making myself stronger in the process.

And this isn't just about cross-cultural conflict. It applies at the personal level, too. My mother and I were family. I was born of her, meaning she was part of me and I of her. But she was also a completely different individual. She had ideas, beliefs, and values that differed from mine—often sharply. But rejecting her outright wouldn't change anything, not in life, and especially not in death. Bottling up my anger might deflect the problems, but it wouldn't solve them. Nor would raging against her, or the memory of her. That cacophony would deepen the hurt all the more. No, I had to find a way to bring her on board, in some way.

IT WASN'T UNTIL I BEGAN TRAVELING ABROAD THAT I EN-countered people who truly believed that their religion was "true" and others "false." The absoluteness of the boundaries between faiths really threw me for a loop. Religious tolerance is a good thing, of course. But the Seven Gods of Happiness show that there are realms beyond tolerance, where differences are celebrated with actual open affection, in the same way we celebrate the differences and quirks of old friends. This is spirituality as a service rather than an obligation or identity, one that encourages interaction with faith traditions for the satisfaction and even joy of the participants, rather than for the faiths themselves.

There's an old saying in Japanese that goes "iwashi no atama mo shinjin kara," which means "to the faithful, even an old sardine head can be divine." It is both serious and satirical: serious in recognizing that even the most humdrum of things can become an object of faith, and satirical in just how humdrum said things might be.

It's especially true in Japan, where the spiritual tendency is to add rather than to refute or negate—there's no "false" when everything's "true." As the folklorist Noboru Miyata put it in a book whose title translated is *The Many Little Kami of Edo*, "The fun of creating kami is at the heart of Japanese folk beliefs . . . We have no problem creating more when needed. That this might be rude to the other kami doesn't even occur to us. When our heads hurt we create kami of headaches; when we suffer from hemorrhoids, kami of hemorrhoids; when our teeth ache, kami of toothaches . . . It's a national characteristic." This propensity for integrating, remixing, and creating totally new spiritual beliefs is precisely why we have such a hard time articulating what we "are" to people from societies where the lines between faiths are far less abstract.

The lines between Shinto and Buddhism can be blurry, but there's another tradition in Japan that takes this kind of spiritual mixing to a different level altogether. Average folks interact with kami and hotoke in shrines and temples and home altars, which is to say in the everyday human world. But there is a group who prefer to meet deities on their own sacred ground, leaving the human realm in search of the divine. The idea is to make contact with higher beings of all sorts so as to gain power—not for themselves but for the purposes of helping other people. They trek deep into the wilderness and subject themselves to trials of physical and mental endurance, both to express their awe at the forces of nature, and in hopes of transcending the human experience to attain a measure of enlightenment. This might sound occult or even a little scary. But it represents one of Japan's oldest spiritual traditions, and one toward which I came to feel a powerful affinity. It's called Shugendo, and learning about it requires a trip deep into the mountains.

CHAPTER 3

Making Friends with Monsters: Shugendo

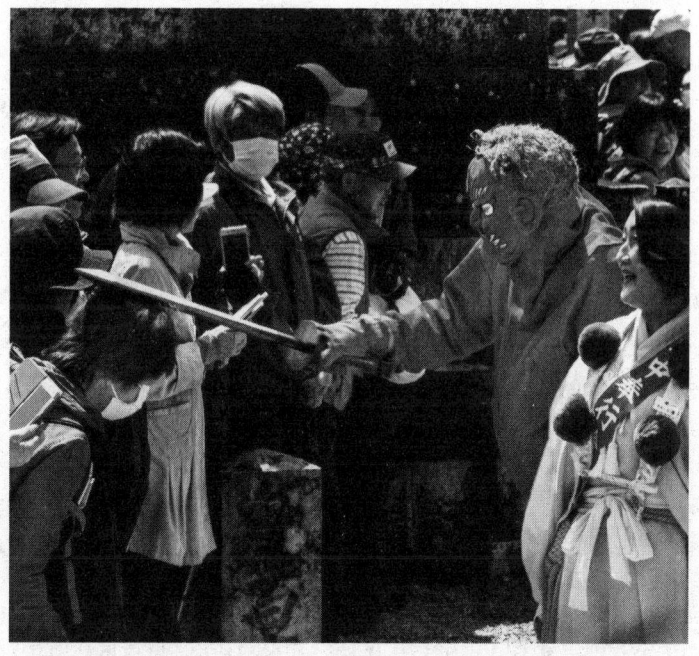

Oni driving out misfortune from visitors at Kinpuseji temple in Nara.
(This particular person asked for relief from hay fever.)

*Everyone, at some point in their lives, has their own time
in the mountains.
Whether you face it with a smile or a frown is up to you.*

—Ryojun Shionuma

*I never visit a shrine for New Year's. I can't believe the kami are
inside those gaudy shrines. It seems much more likely to me that the
kami of the Japanese are deep in the distant mountains and valleys.*

—Hayao Miyazaki

Even when I was very little, ghosts and monsters never intimidated me. Quite the contrary. I was drawn to them. Japanese folklore is filled with all sorts of spooks and creepy-crawlies that we collectively call yokai. They're invisible, like kami—at least in real life. In the collective imagination, it's a different story. Yokai pop up all the time in myths and legends: mischievous and mercurial, sometimes helpful, other times not, but always a signifier of strange happenings. There are many kinds of yokai, and you can often spot them in old artworks, parading across illustrated screens or scrolls or woodblock prints.

My first encounter with a monster, in a manner of speaking, happened in first grade. At the back of my classroom stood a low shelf, sized for children, with many colorful books. One day a new one appeared. Its cover featured a drawing of a round-faced little child. He looked about my age, but his complexion was as white as a sheet, and he seemed not to have any feet. Behind him, almost embracing him, sat a smiling giant, equally pale, proportions as puffy as a marshmallow. Above them was a strange title: *Little Obaké and Muwa-muwa-mu.*

Obaké is a little kid's term for any kind of scary presence (I should note that words like *obaké* and *yokai* shouldn't be confused with *kaiju*, which is used exclusively for giant creatures from film and television, like Godzilla.) And *muwa-muwa* is fluffy-sounding onomatopoeia for wafting clouds or escaping steam. So Muwa-muwa-mu seemed to be the giant's name. That led me to conclude that the boy was Little Obaké. As I began to read, I learned that he was the child of a papa ghost and a mama ghost who lived deep in a forest, and he wanted nothing more than to make new friends. He was a polite little specter, with a unique way of greeting. He would smile, put both hands on his chest, bow, and say: "Good evening! I am not a kaiju. I'm Little Obaké. Say hi to a cat." Only it wasn't evening, he wasn't anything remotely kaiju-like, and there was no cat anywhere to be seen. The randomness of it made me giggle.

Reading the book quickly became part of my daily routine, particularly the section where Obaké introduces himself. "Good evening," I'd recite, practicing greeting a ghost myself. "I am not a kaiju. I'm Hiroko. Say hi to a cat." Between my playing grave with shoeboxes and this new catchphrase, my parents really must have been scratching their heads.

Like many Japanese, I first learned about yokai from cartoons. In the mid-seventies, an anime called *GeGeGe no Kitaro* captivated kids of my generation. As the *Shrek* films would do for Western folklore decades later, it fashioned a patchwork of mythical creatures from different fairy tales into an animated adventure series. I still remember the opening theme, which tantalizingly sang that yokai "don't have to take tests or go to school." It featured a whole cavalcade of strange beings that lurked just beyond the fringes of human perception, with whom only the half-yokai, half-human protagonist Kitaro could interact, an avatar for all of us watching excitedly from our living rooms. He looked like a little kid, but with his wizened expression, tousled hair, bumblebee-striped jacket, and old-fashioned wooden geta sandals, he stood astride worlds: old traditions and modernity, reality and mysterious realms beyond. For a girl who deliberately peered inside closets and under beds in hopes of encountering a yokai or portal into their wonderland, Kitaro was a hero, even a role model.

It was around this time that my classmates and I were gripped by a fad for strange creatures that supposedly stalked small children like ourselves. What started this fad, nobody really knows, but the idea that these *things* were out there went absolutely viral among us kids. The most famous of these spooks was a yokai called Kuchisake-onna, the Slash-Mouthed Woman. The rumors differed from place to place but always unfolded along the same lines. She looks like a normal woman, but she wears a gauze mask . . . *And under that mask her mouth is gruesomely slashed open ear to ear!* She comes up to you wearing the mask, and asks if you think she's pretty. If you say no, she whips out a huge knife and gets you! If you say yes, she rips off her mask to show her ruined mouth, says, "Even like this?" and slashes your face wide open, too! You can't run! 'Cause she can do the hundred-meter dash in three seconds flat! And besides, she has a Lamborghini. What color? Bright red! *Duh!* So went the schoolyard whisper network. Actually, that isn't right. There was nothing whispered—we loved screaming about it.

MY MOTHER SPENT THE LAST FEW YEARS OF HER LIFE ON A sofa in front of the television. The only times she moved were when she woke up in the morning, went to the bathroom, ate at the dining table, or went to bed. She was still ambulatory, but only barely, for walking was risky. My father paid to have the entire house outfitted with handrails, but she would still inevitably lose her balance and fall on a daily basis. I once heard a crash and rushed over to find her on her side in the hallway, next to a small hole she'd knocked through the drywall with her head. It was a miracle she wasn't hurt. We were constantly worried she'd injure herself, yet we also knew that if we restricted her movement, she'd lose what little remaining muscle tone she had. Once that happened, she'd be bedridden. The bathroom and dining table were only about ten steps from the couch, but we figured the risk of that little exercise was worth it.

While sitting in front of the TV was the safest unsupervised activity for her, it came with its own dangers. At some point I noticed that she'd even stopped changing television channels. She wasn't really watching anymore, just staring. When I spoke to her, she had a harder and harder time articulating herself. Her sentences grew progressively shorter. It was obvious that she was losing her mental faculties.

One afternoon, she was acting more strangely than usual. I'd thought she was sleeping, for her head lay back on the headrest. But when I got closer, I saw her hands were in motion. They circled in rhythmic patterns in the air, fluttering above the towel I'd placed on her lap to catch spills. Her eyes were squinted shut in apparent concentration. It reminded me a little of an orchestra conductor, so my first instinct was that she must be thinking about some old favorite song.

"You seem to be enjoying yourself," I said. "What are you doing?"

She opened her eyes and looked at me with a smile.

"Sewing."

I assumed I misheard, and asked her again what she was doing.

"Sewing," she repeated. "But I'm having a hard time. Can you finish it up for me?" She handed me the towel. I looked her in the eye. It was obvious this was no joke: She really thought she was sewing.

Now, I think, I could have played along. I could have taken the towel, agreed to finish the "sewing," and walked away. But I was too young, too shocked, too inexperienced at dealing with a mind in decline, let alone my own mother's. That made accepting the reality of the situation even more difficult. I snapped.

"You aren't sewing! Look, you don't even have a needle in your hand," I said, a little too loudly. My hope was to "wake her up," bring her back to "normal." But it didn't have the intended effect. Her smile crumbled. She didn't say anything—she didn't speak again that night—but her disappointment was palpable. It stung me then, and still does when I think back on it now. At the time, I thought she was simply mad at her daughter, refusing to help in this imaginary chore. But looking back, I think she was more disappointed in herself. My words, intended to help, served only to remind her of her deficits.

A few days later I returned to my parents' house. My mother was hunched over, furiously writing something on a piece of paper. Somehow, I knew it wasn't a letter. Her motions were rapid, practically frantic. I approached her.

In her right hand she clutched a ballpoint pen, and with it she was writing her name over and over again on a blank sheet of printer paper. She'd filled it almost top to bottom. Suddenly she stopped writing and looked at me. I wished she would say something, anything, but she didn't. The silence frightened me. I was still so invested in pretending everything was normal. So I just told her dinner was ready, and helped her to the table. We ate together, the quiet punctuated by my aggressively upbeat comments about the food and weather, anything to try and make a connection.

It wasn't until after I'd gotten her into bed for the night that I looked at the piece of paper again. What I saw sent a chill down my spine. It wasn't just the obsessive density of seeing her name over and over. It was how many of the repetitions were wrong. Some of the kanji-characters had extra or missing strokes. Many more weren't even legible at all, just rickety assemblages of scribbles. I flipped the sheet over. The names continued on the back side, even further devolved. Now they weren't in the complicated kanji characters at all but simple hiragana, the basic phonetic script every child learns in kindergarten. Toward the bottom of the page many of the names weren't even complete. Just her married name, *Yoda . . . Yoda . . . Yoda . . .* over and over. The unfinished repetitions only deepened the sense of horror.

With trembling hands I tore the sheet in two, again and again, using all my force as the overlapping shreds grew thicker and tinier, raining into the trash can next to the desk as though I were trying to erase the evidence of what had happened. What *was* happening.

Looking back on it now, I know my mother must have been even more terrified than I was. After all, I was the healthy one. She was the one going through it. The doctors struggled to define her illness, but its progression was relentless, shrinking her cerebellum and robbing her of her ability to walk, talk, and think. Along the way she began experiencing hallucinations. I clearly remember the first one, because it chilled me to the core.

It happened at night. We were alone that evening, just my mother and I. She emerged from the bathroom, made a beeline for where I was sitting at the kitchen table, grabbed my arm, and said urgently, "Go check the bathroom. Now." Her tone of voice frightened me. I feared a medical emergency of some kind. But when I asked her why, the answer was even more shocking.

"There's a little girl in the bathroom. Yoshiko. She's chanting a sutra in front of the toilet."

The response caught me totally off guard. Yet I could tell she was entirely serious. *This is it*, I thought. *She's finally falling apart.*

Then I realized how silly it all was. A girl reciting Buddhist scripture in front of the commode? And not just any girl, one named Yoshiko? I didn't know any Yoshikos, and I suspected neither did my mother. *Who the heck was she?*

I burst out laughing. "Don't talk like that! You sound like you saw a yokai!"

When my mother's breaks with reality began, many years had passed since my schoolyard fun with Little Obaké and the Slash-Mouthed Woman. But here was another yokai, bubbling up again out of the darkness of my mother's decline. I neither expressed doubt nor professed belief in the strange sutra-chanting girl that my mother saw. Characterizing mother's apparition as a silly yokai, rather than a scary example of mental decay, helped transform an upsetting moment into a lighthearted one.

In a sense, Yoshiko offered a form of salvation. "She" was so absurd, so beyond reason, that she actually made me laugh. A little girl chanting sutras over the toilet bowl? As I laughed, my mother began laughing along with me. And in that moment, that shared moment, things were normal for an instant, mother and daughter enjoying an inside joke.

I told my sister about Yoshiko, and she began invoking her name whenever my mother did or said something inexplicable, such as when we found her calling up the darkened stairs to the second floor in search of a little girl who wasn't there. *It's just Yoshiko again*, we'd chuckle to ourselves. That little poltergeist proved a potent coping mechanism in helping us overcome our fear—our knowledge—of the inexorable progression of our mother's illness. Because the facts of that undeniable transformation were too dark for us to bear. This is what yokai always were and always will be: the faces of things utterly beyond our control, making hard truths more approachable, making dark situations more navigable.

As I write these words, I'm reminded of how darkness inevitably has negative connotations in English. In the West it is associated with chaos, with death and demons, places where evildoers lurk. "No light, but rather darkness visible" is how Milton described Hell in *Paradise Lost*. But Japan has traditionally had more ambivalent feelings about the concept. As Jun'ichiro Tanizaki wrote in his *In Praise of Shadows*, in Japan "darkness causes us no discontent; we resign ourselves to it as inevitable. If light is scarce then light is scarce; we will immerse ourselves in the darkness and there discover its own particular beauty."

"Westerners tend to think of light and dark in opposition," said the director Hayao Miyazaki in a 1988 interview for his celebrated anime film *My Neighbor Totoro*. "But I don't think things can be treated with that kind of duality. For Japanese, the kami are in the darkness. They may come out into the light at times, but they are usually deep in the forest or mountains . . . A sense of awe at the darkness underlies the veneration Japanese have towards certain forests and natural things."

Satsuki and Mei, the sibling protagonists of *My Neighbor Totoro*, has a sick mother, too. At one point her condition takes a terrible turn, and Mei runs off trying to find the hospital on her own, getting terribly lost in the process. Satsuki is overwhelmed by grief over her mother and possibly having lost her baby sister, too. But just when things seem darkest, Totoro, a mysterious creature whom the girls have befriended deep in the shadows of an ancient forest, emerges to help.

Miyazaki's masterwork is a cartoon, of course. Totoro is a figment of his exquisite imagination, never explicitly defined as kami or yokai, or anything other than a Totoro, whatever that might be. But there is truth in this beautiful fiction. Everyone, at some point, will find themselves in the darkness. Yet even in that darkness, there are helpers, if we know how to find them, forces we can tap to assuage our anxieties, to quench our fears, to help us navigate our way through. In Japan's spiritual traditions, darkness can even help one grow.

....

SHINTO AND BUDDHISM ARE JAPAN'S BEST-KNOWN SOURCES of spirituality. But the third tradition, Shugendo, much less talked about but no less influential, is a form of spirituality rooted in the mountains, nourished by all of their beauty and awe, reared in their peaks and valleys, fueled by their hazards and dangers, reveling in their light and shadows. It borrows liberally from Shinto and Buddhism but isn't beholden to either. One can be a practitioner of Shugendo and of Shinto or Buddhism, or both, or neither. This makes it incredibly difficult to explain to outsiders.

Perhaps this is because "Buddhism and Shinto represented the 'front,' while Shugendo magic dealt with the rear, the reversed, the backward, and so forth," as the Shinto scholar Helen Hardacre put it. Practitioners weren't ordained priests or monks but rather outsiders and iconoclasts, living with one foot in the sacred and the other in the profane material world. They eschewed all the comforts and perks of mainstream religion, embracing a rougher path, taking sustenance from hardship and trials. This led to a lot of misconceptions; when Jesuit missionaries first encountered Shugendo in the sixteenth century, they mistook it for devil worship. They were wrong, of course. But it's true that Shugendo practitioners worship deities different from those typically pacified by shrines or temples. Theirs are untamed and unpredictable. Theirs are the wild gods.

The lives of ancient Japanese were yoked to the whims and rhythms of the wild. To them, mountains were more than terrain. Previous generations had tamed the flatlands. But the peaks were beyond human control. They were both the source of the waters that nourished life and the portals to realms unknown to mere mortals. "In the depths of certain mountains, the legends and place-names testified to an ancient belief in paradise," wrote the anthropologist Carmen Blacker in her 1975 survey of Japanese shamanistic beliefs, *The Catalpa Bow*. "In certain valleys vestiges of entrances to hell were to be discovered in the pools of hot mud which bubbled up from sulfur springs. In some of these mountains there must have existed 'another world' even older than the Buddhist heavens and hells, for it was from these steep wooded slopes, which leapt up so precipitously from flat green rice fields, that the ancestral dead were believed to return for the annual visit to their old homes. In yet other holy hills the supernatural denizens were not the dead, but the mysterious numina known as kami."

Every village had its own legends and superstitions about

"Yama-no-kami," the Kami of the Mountain. In the northern reaches, for instance, it was forbidden to enter the mountains on December 12. That was the date of the deity's birth long, long ago, and she—almost always a she, a symbol of fertility, a creator of life—spent that day counting all the trees in her realm. Should a human have the misfortune of being there, they would be "counted" as part of the forest, never allowed to return. And she was believed to be a jealous kami, so women were strongly discouraged from entering the mountains at all, lest they offend with their presence. So the stories went.

This same aura of mysticism and danger also attracted spiritual seekers. They saw the hazards of the highlands as things not to be avoided but to be embraced, in service of transcending the limits of human body and mind. Training is how one obtains (shu) spiritual powers (gen). This is the Way (do). Thus *Shugendo*. Practitioners call themselves "yamabushi"—"those who surrender to the mountains." Yamabushi might climb savage peaks subsisting on nothing but herbs and nuts, recite mantras for long periods in the inky depths of caves, or chant sutras beneath the icy hammer of an alpine waterfall. This isn't idle machismo; their goals are catharsis and purification, proving themselves worthy of contact with the divine, and through that contact, borrowing some of its holy power. For the yamabushi, going into the mountains is a trip in literal and metaphoric senses—a pilgrimage into the wilds, a sacrament in a visionary journey to another plane of existence.

A man named Ryojun Shionuma is one of only a few yamabushi known to have completed the harshest trial of all, called the Thousand Days of Training. The reason so few commit to this ritual is because it means putting their life on the line: Once one begins a walk, it is said, they cannot stop for any reason—not weather, not injury, not sickness. In a 2007 book, he described a regimen of awakening before midnight, standing beneath a waterfall to purify body and soul, then traveling on foot from Kinpusenji to Omine and back. That's thirty-one miles through the mountains in a single day, fortified by only rice balls and water. (Consider that a marathon is "only" 26.2 miles, and that over flat terrain; Shionuma's course took him 4,500 feet up and back again.) He then repeated this process another 999 times over the course of nine years. He wrote of walking amid storm winds that blew hard enough to send fully grown trees flying. He faced physical dangers such as rockfalls and dangerous animals such as snakes, boars, and bears. And he faced inner demons, such as the monsters he hallucinated were throwing rocks at him as he walked in a delirium of exhaustion. And when Shionuma finished—walking 30,969 miles in all; Earth's circumference is only 24,901!—he spent nine days in deep prayer with no food, no drink, and no rest, chanting sutras over and over again. The experience was so intense that his fellow yamabushi held a "living funeral" ceremony for him before the final stretch of prayer.

This sort of thing is extreme even for yamabushi. But when they returned from their trials, whatever they were, the yamabushi traditionally put the skills learned on the "other side" to work here in the material world. History abounds with tales of yamabushi employed as medicinal and faith healers, and as fortune-tellers. They performed exorcisms and purification rituals, and even adjudicated disputes. The abbots of mainstream Buddhist temples and the priests of Shinto shrines tended to inherit their positions along family lines. But there were no such requirements for yamabushi. They occupied a position outside the religious establishment, allowing them to slip into and through and between Shinto and Buddhist traditions with ease, living embodiments of Japan's flexibility in matters of faith. That people of old so respected these outsiders is a sign of our connection to the mountain realms, and to our belief in them as other worlds.

If all this sounds a little mystical, you aren't alone. The sight of yamabushi mountain-shamans in their distinctive garb, so different from that of priest, monk, or average citizen, sent people of yore into flights of fancy. Foreigners projected fantasies of satanic witchcraft. Japanese people conflated man with monster: the tengu, winged giants of mountain folklore. Tengu are yokai, as muscular as bodybuilders, with crimson skin and elongated noses, or blue skin with the heads of ravens, but in either case inevitably clad in the vestments of the yamabushi. Mercurial as the mountains themselves, tengu might take those who showed respect under their wing, while ferociously punishing the discourteous. If someone went missing from a village, it might be said they were "tengu-kakushi"—spirited away by a tengu.

....

THE FIRST TIME I EVER SAW A YAMABUSHI OUTSIDE THE pages of a history book was in the spring of 2009. The occasion was a fire-walking festival at Mount Takao. It was open to the public, in fact widely advertised, and I'd been intrigued enough to go.

When Buddhist monks established a monastery on the slopes of Mount Takao some 1,300 years ago, this was untamed wilderness. Today it is not. A combination of proximity to Tokyo—just an hour's train ride—and ease of hiking make it a popular day trip for city folk and tourists. Gently sloping paths are supplemented by a chairlift and a funicular railroad, making it a breeze for almost anyone to summit, and numerous teahouses and soba shops vending bowls of handmade buckwheat noodles in steaming broth ensure nobody goes hungry. There's even a beer garden halfway up. By some measures, it is the single most climbed mountain in the world. The Michelin Guide gave it three stars back in 2007.

I knew Mount Takao well, as I'd climbed it many times. The very first was on an elementary school field trip. The trail up the mountain takes hikers through the precincts of a temple called Yakuo-in. Its main hall is a glorious structure of unfinished wood, with a sloping copper roof overhanging intricate carvings of mythical animals, its entrance flanked by a pair of giant-size tengu masks. Our teacher told us it was a Buddhist temple.

Many years later I started noticing something was different about Yakuo-in—that the atmosphere there contrasted subtly with other Buddhist temples that I had seen. For one thing, a gorgeous, scarlet-framed Shinto shrine sits up the hill just a few dozen steps above the temple. Now, as I've mentioned, it isn't uncommon for temples to host small shrines on their grounds. But Yakuo-in's shrine is huge, almost as large as, and if anything even more elaborate than, the main hall. Then there are the statues. Portrayals of tengu are everywhere on the grounds, some human-size, some much larger, their muscular bodies rendered in weathered bronze, standing near entrance ways as guardians, arms and swords raised. But most surprising of all is the deity venerated inside Yakuo-in. The Buddhist statuary I knew generally had gentle appearances, but here on Mount Takao the monks worshipped a ferocious-looking entity called Izuna Daigongen: the Great Avatar of Izuna.

A massive, larger-than-human statue stood behind the altar of Yakuo-in prayer hall, raven-like face drawn into a fierce grimace, body wreathed in flames, a sword held at the ready in one hand and a coiled rope in the other. Later I would learn it represented aspects of five Buddhist deities merged into a single kami, and it was posed standing atop a white fox, the stereotypical animal-familiar of Japanese lore. Unsurprisingly, warlords of old worshipped this deity in hopes of righteous victory. Yet in spite of its startling appearance, the Great Avatar of Izuna is a protector and even bringer of happiness to those who pay their respects. This duality, ferocity and benevolence personified in a single powerful package, is a signature of this religious practice. Yakuo-in is a temple, but not a Buddhist one, or not exactly. It is a Shugendo temple. Which is to say, Mount Takao, Michelin stars and all, is a Shugendo mountain, a place where, long ago when this was a far less tame place than it is now, seekers forged into wilderness in search of wisdom.

Fire, like the conflagration enveloping the Great Avatar of Izuna, is key to Shugendo and esoteric Buddhist rituals both. In religious ceremonies, it serves to burn away misfortune and impurities. But only the yamabushi perform public "demonstrations of the magic art, undertaken to convince the community that the disciple has indeed risen above the ordinary human state," Carmen Blacker wrote "Until the end of the 19th century a fair number of these feats could still be witnessed in various parts of Japan. Today the repertory seems to have been reduced to three: *hi-watari* or fire walking, *yudate* or sousing oneself in boiling water, and more rarely *katana-watari* or climbing up a ladder of swords."

On the day of the firewalk, the yamabushi had prepared a large field at the base of the mountain, flat and open, without any trees or buildings around. I'd soon understand why.

In the middle of the clearing stood an enormous mound of cypress boughs collected from the forest, a giant rectangle easily thirty feet long, and a good seven feet high. I arrived early to get a front-row view, and I was glad I did, for in the hours leading up to the ceremony, the viewing area filled with hundreds and hundreds of onlookers as curious as I was, pushing me up against the ropes that had been hung to keep us civilians from getting too close to what was about to happen.

Suddenly the sound of conch-shell horns rippled through the air, deep and resonant, heralding the entrance of nearly a hundred yamabushi into the ceremonial area. Over the next hour or so, they took turns performing a variety of purification rituals. One dipped a large whisk fashioned out of bamboo leaves into a cauldron of boiling water, then whipped the scalding branches over his shoulders over and over again. Another swung a ceremonial sword in abstract patterns designed to sever links to evil entities. Another fired arrows from a longbow into the corners of the mound of cypress to create a kekkai, a sacred field. And finally, after making their preparations, the yamabushi used torches to light the pyre of boughs.

The flames raced sideways along the densely stacked branches like foxes leaping across a hillside, trailing sparks that increased in size as they reached upward and upward. It was a fair but breezy day. A sudden gust seized those threads of fire and unified them into a singular massive pillar of flame that rose into the sky like a red dragon. It was as though the fire had consumed the mountains beyond and might catch the sky on fire.

The heat radiating from the pyre was substantial, physical, a pressure you could feel. I couldn't imagine being any closer than I was, yet several yamabushi ran to and fro just footsteps from the conflagration. With wooden buckets they doused its base to keep it under control, faces beet red from proximity to the heat. Several fire trucks also stood at the ready, just in case. Occasionally the pyre would belch a cloud of sparks into the air that flitted about and drifted down like literal fireflies; later that night, at home, I would notice several tiny holes burned into my new winter jacket.

The fire was impressive, but the ceremony's finish was even more so. After the boughs had burned into ash, the yamabushi used rakes to spread the embers into what resembled a large glowing carpet. Then they removed their footwear and began to walk. Their first steps were atop a mound of salt, a traditional form of purification. Then one by one they strolled over the embers, still very much alive and smoldering, in bare feet. A line of them crossed, each step planted firmly, resolutely, into the inferno stretching before them. The announcer described this as their way of surrendering evil passions and praying for peace and relief from suffering. Then, once the yamabushi had completed their traversal, the announcer opened the path to anyone who wished to walk. Many spectators did, and so did I. In fact, there were so many people waiting their turn that it took nearly an hour for mine. The ash had cooled by then, but was still very warm.

So went my first experience with yamabushi. The rituals, the trials, the pyre, and the fire walking—all of it so exotic to me. To be honest, they seemed almost superhuman. I wanted to know more. When I studied for my Shinto Cultural Examinations in 2012, I was hoping to learn more about Shugendo as well. But the textbooks touched on the tradition in only the broadest of historical strokes. It gave me valuable context, but it still didn't give me much of an idea of what Shugendo was, or what yamabushi actually did. Shugendo, "the way of acquiring power," sounds as vague in Japanese as it does in English. And as for what the tradition was, well, that changed depending on what point in history you were talking about, what region you were talking about, even what person you were talking about. It was slippery stuff. I knew I was merely touching the surface, and every theory I posed to myself was almost immediately disputed by different information. It felt like the old parable about the blind men describing an elephant, unable to reconcile the limits of their localized experiences with one another.

Yet I was clear about one thing. Shugendo represented the third most influential belief system in Japan, and it remains active today. So why didn't we hear more about it? What ongoing purpose did Shugendo serve in our modern "secular" society? Did their mastery of "magic," as I'd seen at the firewalk, have any relevance for modern folk like me? At first glance the yamabushi, with their archaic robes and their strange traditions, seemed lost in time, superheroes from another era. But that couldn't be right. These had to be people, just like me, and their beliefs had to be grounded in some kind of modern reality.

So I decided I'd participate in a yamabushi training session myself. Maybe that way I might get some answers. I didn't know what form this training would take, but of one thing I was certain: My path led into the mountains.

....

I WASN'T INTERESTED IN AFFILIATING MYSELF WITH ANY particular temple or sect, so I did my best to try out as many Shugendo-like training experiences as I could find. Some were Buddhist-inflected; others, more Shinto-oriented. These generally aren't publicized, but there are quite a few if you start looking for them, or rather listening, through word of mouth.

It was on one of these outings that I first trained beneath

a waterfall, under the watchful eye of a Shinto guide. We were at an elevation of 3,281 feet, and it was November. Dressed in white robes, we entered the basin one by one, spending as much time under the freezing waters as we were able. But this was no test of endurance. It was intended to focus our minds on the moment. This was a relatively small waterfall, in height and flow, but even still, the relentless hammer of icy water could injure if one wasn't careful. Our guide made sure that we positioned ourselves so it fell on our shoulder blades rather than directly on our heads.

At first contact with that icy rain, it felt as though every muscle turned to stone. The sound of thundering water filled my ears, my mind, my soul. Initially, I tried to push back against that relentless pressure, tensing myself to keep myself upright. But I quickly realized that there was no way to "win" against the forces of nature. So I gave up. I let the tension flow from my body as though washed away by the frigid flow. I've often seen this practice described as "meditation" in English, and while I can't speak for everyone who does it, that word doesn't fit my experience at all. It felt like a cleansing or a purification, and a connection to natural forces in a truly visceral, whole-body way.

There were some dramatic moments on the trip. I learned of a monk who would take those who inquired to a prayer hall hidden deep in the mountains. I contacted him, and he agreed to show me. We met in the office of his temple. He was in his early forties, perhaps, with a shaved head and dressed in a linen samue, the workwear of a monk. Together we hiked into the foothills above his temple. After an hour, he announced we had arrived. Before us was a strange sight: a sturdy iron gate, set directly into the steep mountainside. Behind it I could see a natural vestibule and, deeper within it, a small altar of wood on a pedestal of stone.

The monk began reciting sutras, and I followed as best I could. When we finished, he produced a key and unlocked the gate. The chamber where the altar stood seemed at first to be a dead end. But then the monk pointed out metal rungs set into the wall off to one side, all but hidden in shadow. They led to a manhole-size opening in the ceiling, a natural tunnel extending almost vertically up through volcanic stone. He bade me to follow him. As we started to climb, he began chanting sutras once again.

The rungs led to a ladder made of chain, which swayed and clinked as we ascended, the path upward lit by only the feeble flicker of candles placed on holders along the way. We ascended for what felt like a very long time, my only guides the cold metal against my hands and the chanting of the monk above.

Eventually, the monk fell silent. We had reached a small antechamber, perhaps ten feet on a side. But its size belied its majesty, as our candles illuminated pearlescent stalactites shimmering in the haze above like a natural chandelier. The monk resumed his chant. The sutras echoed all around, surrounding us like an aural embrace as we pressed our palms together in the candlelight. Later the monk told me there were chambers beyond, ones he'd never been to himself, where his own master went to perform rituals deep within the mountain itself. I'd never prayed like this before. I may well never pray this way ever again. But I will never forget making this connection to the earth, in a very literal sense. It felt like returning to a womb of earth and stone.

I don't know that I experienced any kind of transcendental awakening through these experiences. I loved the idea of cultivating a positive, can-do attitude to power through hardships and difficulties. I enjoyed fantasizing about what kind of power I might find within myself. I was in fact close to choosing a Shugendo sect, to train for real. I worried about how my husband might take it.

....

AS WITH BUDDHISM, THERE ARE MANY SCHOOLS OF SHU-gendo. I chose the one centered at Kinpusenji Temple, of Nara Prefecture, in the town of Yoshino. I picked it because it represents one of Shugendo's most sacred sites, as its background story is closely associated with the man who is venerated as the founder of Shugendo itself.

His name is En. He was a self-ordained monk who spent most of his time in the wilderness, which is why he is also called En the Unordained and En the Ascetic. En's name is virtually synonymous with "holy man" in Japan, even among laypeople. So is his appearance, as he's a common subject of traditional art and sculpture. Sometimes I think of him as Japan's answer to Gandalf the Grey from *Lord of the Rings*, because he's portrayed as an old mystic in robes and often accompanied by his familiars, a pair of fierce-looking horned ogres.

Statues of En are common sights on sacred ground, not only Shinto shrines and Buddhist temples but also outdoors, particularly on mountains, as he's famed in legend for having climbed peaks all over Japan. Some 70 percent of Japan is covered in mountains, so if you're the sort who enjoys hiking, like I do, there's a high chance of running into an old stone effigy of En.

There's one atop Mount Takao, actually, just inside the first gate of Yakuo-in temple. People leave offerings there of miniature geta, those one-toothed wooden sandals worn by holy mountain men in times of old, in hopes for strong and healthy legs. And Shugendo practitioners have adopted En as a shared guardian spirit, a kind of patron saint. He must have been a rather extraordinary person to have had such a big impact on Japanese spirituality, I thought. And his story, or at least one of them, begins at Kinpusenji temple. So that is where I started my quest.

Kinpusenji is located on Mount Yoshino. Its slopes are covered with tens of thousands of cherry trees, and every spring, tourists flock there to lavish in a sea of pink and white that blankets the entire mountain. Yoshino serves as the entrance to the vast Omine mountain range, and Kinpusenji sits atop it, in a clearing that offers a spectacular view of the peaks all around. There's a statue of En there, too, of course. The sight of it silhouetted against the Omine peaks only reinforced the sense that I was stepping into his spiritual home ground.

Kinpusenji is an unusual sort of place. The temple's main hall has stood on this spot for more than four hundred years. There are many old structures in Japan, but this one is unique, constructed of pillars made from different species of tree. As you walk through the hall's cavernous interior, you find yourself surrounded by columns of cedar, keyaki elm, pine, and tsutsuji azalea. There's even the titanic trunk of what must have been an enormous pear tree, harvested four centuries ago. I'm not a botanist; I know this only because the pillars are labeled, and not simply for historical reference. Kinpusenji's main hall is a place of worship, but it also functions as a sort of virtual reality, a re-creation of a deep forest, primeval and ancient. The hall represents the wilds, where yamabushi sought answers to life's quandaries, in symbolic form: a gathering place for normal folk who couldn't face the trials of the wild themselves.

In the center of the hall sits a massive altar, supporting a trio of enormous statues of an incredibly ferocious-looking deity named Zao Daigongen—the Great Avatar of Zao. The tallest of the three stands well over twenty feet, with indigo blue skin and a wild shock of hair blown back as if by divine wind, wreathed in elaborately carved flame, one foot raised as though about to thunder down on the ground below, one arm raised, grasping a double-ended trident. His left arm is frozen in midair, two fingers extended, capturing a motion symbolizing the swing of a sword. He is flanked by two other manifestations of himself, each slightly shorter but equally impressive. The triad represents Zao Daigongen in the past, present, and future.

For centuries, these dramatic statues were hidden behind titanic doors, off-limits to all but the monks who attended to them. Visitors who prayed at the altar then were obliged to imagine what might lie behind those doors, their awe stoked, no doubt, by the thought of the divine presences that dwelled so close yet out of sight.

So it was, until 2004. That is when UNESCO recognized Kinpusenji as a World Heritage Site along with a number of other holy spots in the region, and the temple decided to open the Zao triad to public display. More recently, the temple has opened the altar doors more regularly, on a handful of special days scattered throughout the year. This is because these statues proved a great draw for tourists, and this in turn helps the monks solicit money for much-needed renovations. Visitors are charged for the privilege of viewing the statues—for it isn't easy or cheap to maintain a temple as old as this one.

When those doors are open, and the avatars loom over you in that "forest" of tree trunks, you are transported to the moment when Zao Daigongen is said to have manifested before a holy man on a hilltop, thirteen centuries ago. That holy man was En the Ascetic.

En was born some thirteen hundred years ago, in a tiny village in rural Nara. He spent his youth studying Buddhism at a local temple. That is where history ends and legend begins.

They say that he dreamed of more than just mastering the sutras, that true enlightenment could be found only by forging one's body and mind in the harsh environment of untamed nature. He left behind the comfort of the temple, turning to caves and the wilderness, where he meditated regardless of season or weather. He dreamed of a rainbow-colored cloud descending to Earth, which might loft him through the skies to the mythical garden palace of the Great Sages, where he might drink of their knowledge and dine on the rarefied mists that sustained them, that he might acquire their holy powers to help all humankind. Some say his dream came true.

En lived through some truly trying times. At one point, Japan was racked by a horrific confluence of famine, earthquake, and plague. Nearly a third of the population perished, and Japan's greatest minds wrestled with how to save their nation.

En took the task upon himself. He headed for the peak of Mount Sanjogatake, where he fasted, prayed, and conducted rituals for a thousand days straight. His singular purpose was to make contact with the most powerful deity he could, in the hopes it might assuage the natural horrors wreaking havoc in the land.

The first to appear before him were a real dream team: Shaka Nyorai, the Buddha himself; Senju Kannon, the thousand-armed female bodhisattva of compassion; and Miroku Bosatsu, an avatar of the Buddha's projected return far in the future.

While En expressed much gratitude for their arrival, he also felt they were too gentle-hearted for the task at hand. So he continued to pray. Eventually, the skies darkened, the earth shook, and lightning ripped through the air. When En looked up, he saw a terrifying sight: Zao Daigongen, his monstrously titanic body topped by a ferociously scowling face that somehow radiated anger, compassion, and forgiveness all at the same time. *This would do*, thought En. A fearsome deity for a monstrous era racked by fearsome adversaries. He carved the image of what he had seen into the bark of a cherry tree, so that he might convey it to others.

So go the stories, which don't seem to have a satisfying ending, in a Western storytelling sense. Did his efforts banish the plague, or restore peace to the beleaguered people? We don't know. But that isn't the point. It's tempting to believe that if you only pray hard enough, a savior will arrive to solve all your problems. But that isn't what the stories tell us. Through subjecting himself to such an ordeal on an inhospitable mountaintop, En attained a form of enlightenment. That power was his to wield, for all of us. The invisibles wouldn't save us. But the human spirit, focused on helping others, might.

After En's death in 701 CE, those inspired by his example carried on, and transmitted his worldview and teachings to their disciples, and so on and so on. Many generations later, these traditions coalesced into what we now know as Shugendo.

At Kinpusenji, I'd found a guidebook for participating in a yamabushi training session. I bought it, took it home, read it, and, following its instructions, sent in a request. "Sent" as in physically mailed. No email, no phone: Only postcards were accepted. We had several back-and-forths by snail mail, ironing out the details of what to bring and wear. All of this culminated in a singular cryptic instruction.

Meet us at Muda Crossing. Look for the willow tree.

This, and the name of a nearby train station, was the only guidance I had. The journey took many hours and many changes of train lines from Tokyo. Eventually, I found myself in a little town about an hour outside of Yoshino on a warm, late-spring morning.

At the station, I'd asked an attendant about Muda Crossing, and they'd pointed the way down a two-lane country road paralleling the tracks. A ten-minute walk through a neighborhood of homes framed in the traditional style, with heavy clay-tiled roofs, brought me to the promised willow tree.

I was surprised to find it small and young, only a little taller than me. Was this the right willow? Next to the willow stood an old stone lantern, marking where a wooden footbridge had once stretched across the Yoshino River, carrying travelers across the waters to the foothills of Mount Yoshino beyond. That old bridge was long gone, replaced by a modern span. Across it I could see hills rolling sumptuously across the horizon.

By this time, I had learned there is almost no such thing as a full-time yamabushi; most of them hold regular jobs and lead everyday lives in between their training sessions. Practice trials like this one are the way the vast majority of modern yamabushi come into the fold.

Participants began to arrive over the next hour. By the time of our scheduled departure, we numbered twenty-eight. We were a motley crew of people from all walks of life, the youngest a fourteen-year-old boy, and the oldest a woman of seventy. Most were here for the first time; others, I gathered, were repeat visitors. Some appeared to be affiliated with religious groups. Here and there I noticed religious sashes known as kesa, strips of bright cloth hung around the neck with the crests of various Buddhist sects. It was yet another example of Shugendo's reach beyond religious borders, how it might be harnessed by anybody to "acquire power."

Three men, obviously yamabushi, arrived to guide us on the trip. I say "obviously" because of how distinctly their regalia stood out against the sea of modern Gore-Tex fabric and hiking gear of the participants. White robes and vestments adorned by what looked like fuzzy pom-poms; deer pelts tied around their waists; traditional two-toed boots on their feet. Atop their heads they wore boxlike hexagonal tokin hats, fastened under their chins with braided cords. And each carried his own conch-shell trumpet, that audio-visual signature of Shugendo.

After welcoming us, the yamabushi arranged us in a line, with one of them taking up the front and two bringing up the rear. I was third from the front, wondering what I'd gotten myself into, when a blast from the conch-shell trumpet sounded, deep and resonant. The note echoed across the river and back, sounding more like the call of some strange animal than a human-made sound. The leader told us they call it the "lion's roar." It had the power to drive away evil spirits of all kinds, including the anxieties in the human heart. In spite of its shockingly loud volume, there was something warm and welcoming about the sound, perhaps because it resonated from the curves of that shell, made by nature rather than the human hand. So cleansed, we began our journey, marching downriver and across the bridge.

No sooner had we crossed the span than we came to a stop. The yamabushi pointed out a statue of En and, with their guidance, led us in a group chant of sutras. Fortunately, I'd picked up a pocket-size book of sutras at Kinpusenji temple beforehand. I quickly dropped my backpack, rustled through to find the booklet, and hastily flipped through to catch up with the sutra they were chanting. Our voices echoed through the streets of a quiet neighborhood filled with low houses. Then we began walking again, following a road that sloped gently upward, taking us on a serpentine path to the foothills above.

We eventually trekked a total of nine miles from our starting point to our destination, Kinpusenji temple. This was the beginning of a longer, roughly sixty-mile traditional pilgrimage route from Yoshino called "the inner path through the great peaks," one of the steepest training routes in all of Shugendo. The segment we spent the day walking was largely paved, but beyond Kinpusenji, we were told, it grows rugged and isolated. A number of particularly demanding sections compelled travelers to navigate narrow paths cutting along steep slopes or scrabble their way up cliff faces.

I run and hike regularly, so nine miles wasn't particularly taxing for me. But some of the other participants were having a tough go of things on the sustained climb. The yamabushi bringing up the rear took special care not to let anyone fall behind. Yet this was no recreational trip, and they exhorted us along. "Push yourself too far without pushing yourself too far," one said in what was meant as encouragement.

There were no instructions or guidance beyond this. The rule was to follow the head yamabushi in contemplative silence. But during a water break, I couldn't resist striking up a conversation with him. I asked what it took to become a yamabushi.

"We're masochists," he laughed. "Really upbeat masochists."

I laughed, too, but pressed for more.

"Let me give you an example," he continued. "If we reach a mountain hut and there aren't enough camping mattresses for everyone, a veteran yamabushi will always let the less experienced ones take them. The more experience you have, the more likely you'll be sleeping on the floor. And if there happen to be warmer and colder spots on the floor, the more experienced yamabushi will gravitate towards the colder ones." He paused for a moment and chuckled. "Ten to one, we'd even be saying, 'Thank you for giving me this cold, hard wooden floor,' out of gratitude for having even that—anything beats sleeping out on the ground in the winter!"

It reminded me of what Ryojin Shionuma described as his trick for making it through his thousand-day trial: "Taking pleasure in the things you can't control." It reminded me of my experience under the waterfall, giving myself over to the freezing waters. The vast majority of us will never experience a pilgrimage of the kinds that yamabushi subject themselves to. But we'll all find ourselves in the metaphorical mountains at some point, and cultivating a roll-with-the-punches attitude is key to making it through.

....

THIS MADE SENSE LOGICALLY, BUT IT'S EASIER SAID THAN done. And soon, I'd be tested myself. It didn't involve sleeping rough, but it certainly represented something I couldn't control. It happened several days after my experience with the yamabushi. Once our walk ended, I'd continued traveling in the region on my own. I planned to end the trip in a special way: at Mount Sanjogatake, the place where Shugendo was born thirteen centuries ago.

I wanted to see the spot where it happened. I wanted to see if I might feel any power for myself. I was ready. I'd come all this way. The gate stood before me. A pair of wooden posts six feet tall, with a board connecting the tops, a rudimentary door framing the wilderness beyond. Beside it stood a stone pillar, rough-hewn and squared, towering even taller than the gate. On it a series of characters were engraved deep into the surface.

女 人 結 界

They meant: *WOMEN FORBIDDEN*.

Shugendo started here, just a few hundred yards from where I stood. I yearned to see it, with all my being. Yet here I was being told I could never tread that path. Not out of any fault of my own. Because of my gender.

As I mentioned, there are many schools of Shugendo. Most accept female trainees, who can go on to become full-fledged yamabushi in their own right. And the Meiji government lifted the prohibition on women entering the mountains in 1872, as part of its efforts to stamp out superstitions and modernize. But local men in a handful of places fought back, demanding that their mountains be allowed to retain the taboo, citing faith and tradition. This was one of them.

I knew this before coming here. When UNESCO recognized the Kii area as a World Heritage Site in 2004, a group of local citizens circulated a petition to allow women access to Sanjogatake. They framed it as a matter of human rights, got a lot of media attention, and collected more than ten thousand signatures in support. But nothing came of the matter, and the mountain remained closed to my gender.

"With religious beliefs, it can be difficult to discern 'tradition' from 'prejudice,'" wrote the religious studies professor Naoko Kobayashi in 2024, lamenting how little progress had been made in the two decades since the petition. "The ones making these decisions are men. Until that is addressed, a true discussion can never happen."

I came nevertheless. I'd felt I needed to. Still, no matter that I expected to encounter them, seeing the actual words banning me from further progress stung.

I stood in silence before the "door." I stood for a very long time. All around me towered enormous cedars, sturdy trunks lofting fragrant boughs to scrape the sky far above. Through the gently swaying canopy I caught snatches of azure sky. The atmosphere was silent and majestic. There was no birdsong, no animal patter atop the needles littering the forest floor. The only sound was the muffled roar of the river behind me, whose translucent-emerald waters I had glimpsed from on high as I'd crossed the final bridge to get here, to the sacred grove at the foot of the sacred mountain. A breeze tousled my hair as I stared down the path beyond the gate.

There was nobody else around. I could have ignored the prohibition and walked through the gateway. I could have summited that peak and nobody would have been the wiser. But I didn't. I came here to show respect, not to challenge taboos. I came because I wanted to get as close as I could, and I had.

The cedars continued to sway overhead. After a while I felt as though they were looking down at me, asking me questions. I could imagine their voices, deep with woody gravitas: *What are you doing here? What do you want?*

I am a feminist. I consider myself a fighter for equality. I know that my nation is behind the times when it comes to the treatment of women. Japan regularly comes in last among the advanced nations in the World Economic Forum's *Global Gender Gap Report*.

I feel this in my bones. When I was a young woman fresh out of college, my nation's sexism drove me to quit my corporate job, to leave a respectable career path, to head back to school in America and start my own business there. My society's tendency to prioritize the desires of men over the needs of women sickened me. More than that—it had literally driven me out of society altogether for a time. A big part of me had never wanted to come back. But I had, and here I was, standing on a mountainside, looking at chauvinism carved into cold, hard stone.

Normally, whenever I think about this kind of thing, it makes the bile rise. But there on Sanjogatake, for some reason, I felt cold reason. I'd been trying to learn something from Shugendo, and I had, from my experiences with the yamabushi. They had taken me in, allowed me to train with them. I could continue that training if I so desired. Shugendo wasn't the problem. Sexism masquerading as tradition was. Shugendo had changed. This place hadn't.

But at the same time, a poem popped into my head. It was written by Jikigyo Miroku, a spiritual seeker who founded a popular religious sect that worshipped Mount Fuji, early in the eighteenth century.

One climbs Mt. Fuji
and finds nothing there
whether that is good or bad
is in one's mind

Summiting Mount Sanjogatake wouldn't solve anything. It wouldn't answer any questions. It would be as much "nothing there" as up on Fuji, or anywhere. The only real answers lay within.

I AM NOT A YAMABUSHI. BUT I LOVE THE MOUNTAINS. AND the fact is, climbing a peak isn't the only way to appreciate its beauty. Japan is so mountainous that it's rare to be far from the sight of one. Mount Fuji, our tallest, is a perfect example. I was born and raised in Tokyo. Mount Fuji is almost sixty miles distant. Yet it's easy to spot that elegantly sloped, almost perfectly symmetrical peak here and there, between houses and high-rises, off in the distance, particularly in the cold, clear air of winter. There are actually many place-names in Tokyo named for their views of Fuji, such as Fujimidai, literally "Fuji-view heights." When I commuted to school as a little girl, catching sight of that snowcapped peak through a tiny slit of space between a noodle shop and the fence of the train station in my neighborhood always made my day, as though I'd captured a tiny but measurable bit of good luck. Many years have passed since those days, but I feel the same attachment to Mount Fuji. Every time I see it inside (and of course outside) of Tokyo, it brightens my day.

When I was eleven, my parents took me on a trip to climb Mount Fuji. On the way up, I came down with a terrible case of altitude sickness, and we had to turn back. I've since learned that some people are simply more susceptible to it than others; it comes down to genetics. But even though I never made it to the top, Mount Fuji lost nothing of its charm to me. Now I'd approached another peak I'd always wanted to climb, and found myself turned back again.

I recalled another story about En the Aesthetic. Late in life, they say, he encountered a pair of oni—ferocious ogres—deep in the mountains. Normal people would have run in terror, and probably been devoured for their troubles. But not En. Through his mastery of the mystical arts, he compelled them to renounce their evil ways and become his disciples. Virtually every portrayal of En in art shows him flanked by these two fearsome monsters. "Should they disobey him," says *Shoku Nihongi*, an official history of Japan commissioned by the emperor in the eighth century, "he would bind them with spells. But he used them to gather his firewood and fetch his water."

The idea of En harnessing these frightening monsters for the purposes of housekeeping, rather than for taking power or causing mayhem, seems amusing, even a little cute. But I think it teaches us something important: that our monsters can't be erased or banished; they will always be with us. Yet if we face them with the right mindset, they can be tamed. They can even help us in our daily lives.

"You will face different trials every time you train," says the yamabushi Kokai Shimazu. "But the most difficult trial of them all is facing yourself." I wasn't even standing on the mountain's training ground at that moment. Yet I felt the mountain taught me something nonetheless. When I faced Sanjogatake, it sparked an awareness of my true feelings: negative, even angry ones. These were my inner demons, monsters who menaced my thinking. But I did not run from them. I did not get eaten. I faced them, and like En, embraced them and tamed them. Whether I could use them like he could, I didn't know. But it was a start. I am a woman. Whether I see that as a hindrance or a strength is up to me. And if that is my choice, I choose strength.

....

MOUNTAINS ARE A TERRAIN, BUT THEY ARE ALSO A META-phor. They symbolize the hardships we face in our lives. This is the story that the architects of the great hall of Kinpusenji, itself a facsimile of a mountain wilderness, have encoded within the structure they built four centuries ago.

But the real mountains are inside us. My mother's deterioration was a mountain I found myself forced to climb, one whose peak I could never summit, nor find answers on. It was just putting one foot in front of the other, day by day.

When she was still healthy, my mother sometimes told me about her own mother's end, and her regret over how she'd dealt with it. On her deathbed, my grandmother began speaking of a cloud floating around her. She desperately wanted to ride it but was too weak to get out of bed. She begged my mother to help. *Was it rainbow-colored like En's?* I wonder now, as I recall this long-ago story. *Would she find her own parents and grandparents, gone so many years, waiting in the gardens of the heavens?*

My mother was then only twenty-three years old, even younger than I was when I faced her decline. "There is no cloud," she told my grandmother. "You're imagining things." She said my grandmother's face fell when she heard this. That disappointment, that sadness, etched itself deep into my mother's heart.

"I should have played along with her," she'd tell me. "I should have played along." She brought it up many times when I was young. I suspect she carried it with her to her own end.

But I was too young to understand when I first heard this sad story. It was only much later, after the "sewing" incident, that I remembered. I still regret not playing along with my mother that evening. The memory still stings, even now, as I write about it. But unlike my mother, I had a second chance in the form of the little girl Yoshiko. She appeared deep in the wilderness of my mother's decline. Looking back, perhaps I actually had gone through a trial of my own, not on a physical mountain but a metaphorical one, standing by my mother through that long, sad process of deterioration and disintegration. Perhaps that gave me the strength to transform a dark moment into a helpful monster in the form of Yoshiko. I am eternally grateful to her for popping out of the darkness to guide us through those last trying days. Monsters are a metaphor, too, and they come in all shapes and sizes.

Yamabushi literally means "those who surrender to the mountains." But what it really means, I think, is to acknowledge that we are but small pieces in the unfathomably large puzzle that is life. Yamabushi or not, we share that, one and all. The yamabushi found their gen, their power, through their trials in the darkness of their mountains. And I found my gen in the darkness of mine, in the trials of my mother's illness.

Looking back, I think that is what gave me the power to reengage with Japan's spiritual traditions in the first place. Along the way, I learned a great deal about the fundamental belief systems underlying my own culture, from Shinto to Buddhism to Shugendo. That process of learning proved more than educational: It nourished and healed. One of the most important lessons was that kami and hotoke can be found everywhere. When I found myself at a truly dark point in my life, finding "helpers" even in the midst of it, closer to me than I ever imagined, was more than helpful. It was empowering. That realization was valuable enough in and of itself. But as it turned out, it would also prove an asset in more personal trials that I would soon face.

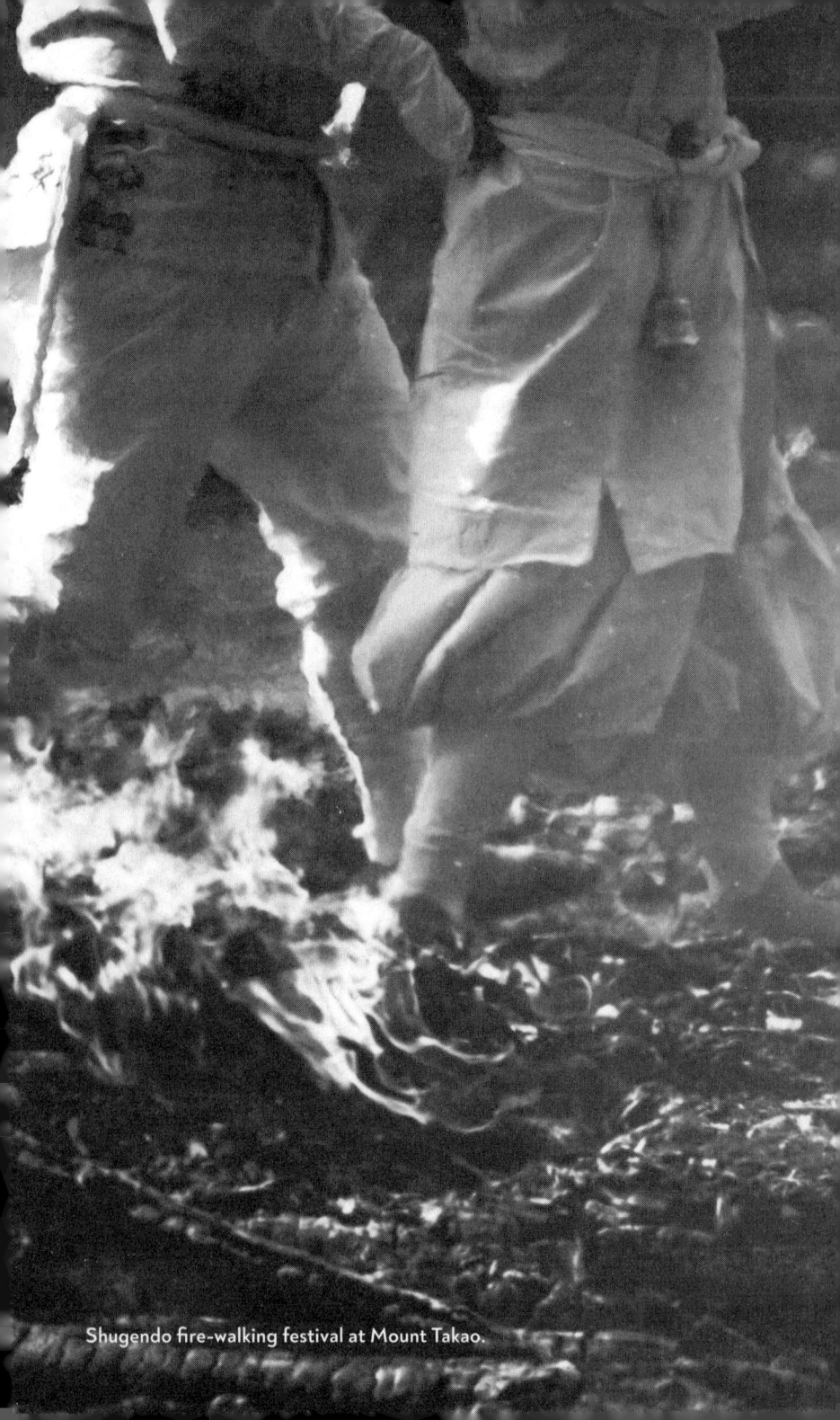

Shugendo fire-walking festival at Mount Takao.

Part Two

DARKNESS: WALKING THROUGH HARDSHIP

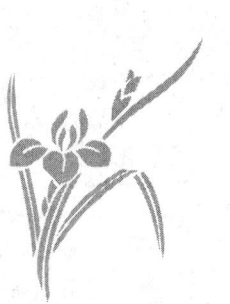

CHAPTER 4

Angry Ghosts: Onryo

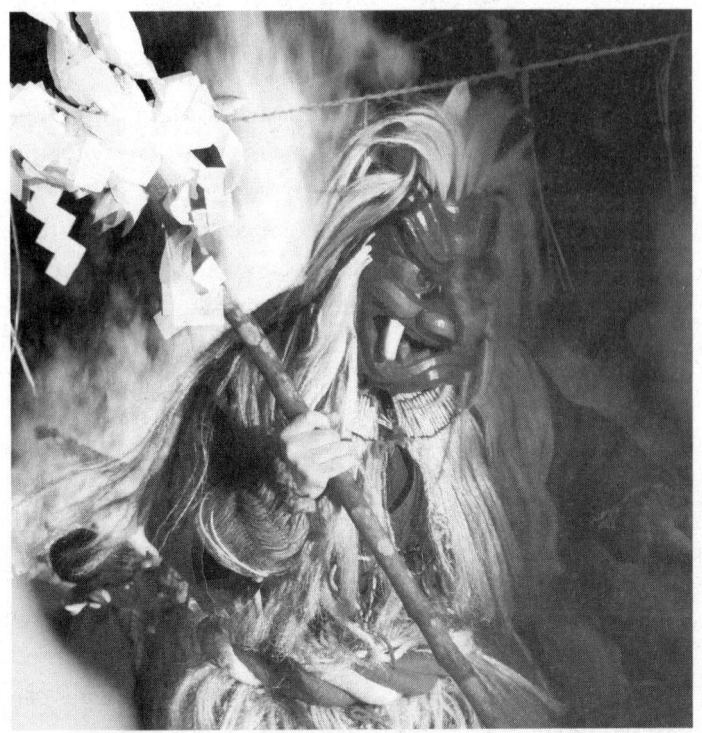

Sedo Matsuri Festival in Akita.

We are all haunted by the "ghosts" of our past selves, selves we left behind as we chose one path over another in the past . . . The necessity of quelling them is what makes us human.

—Noboru Yasuda, Noh performer

Anger comes when I least expect it, in waves large and small, snippets of memory washing over me like ocean tides, throwing me off-balance as the sands of time shift beneath my feet.

It doesn't happen often, but for some reason, it always seems to coincide with my brushing my teeth in the morning. I've come to think of this as my own personal "witching hour," that moment when Western folklore says ghosts are most likely to appear. Perhaps it is because I am still between wake and sleep, the gears of my consciousness only starting to grind back into life. I am relaxed, but also off guard. Sometimes my subconscious chooses this moment to open the floodgates a crack, and out sneak memories that I've tried to consign to the darkness.

My mother compared me with my younger sister endlessly. Anytime I said something wrong, or didn't do something in the way my mother expected, I'd hear: *Your little sister wouldn't do this. Your little sister does that. Why can't you be more like your little sister?* It felt like I had to fight for everything I ever wanted, simply for having been born two years earlier. Looking back now, I see this as her attempt to foster a sense of responsibility in me. But at the time, I hated her for it.

As with so many first children, my parents were always stricter with me. No doubt they saw their instincts as protective, but to me, a little girl at the time, it all felt restrictive and preordained. *Stop it, Hiroko. No, you can't do that. This discussion is over.* Yet, should my little sister attempt the exact same thing, she would be permitted, even encouraged.

One day, out of exasperation, I confronted my mother. Why was everything between us a fight, while my sister got everything she asked for on a silver platter? I can hear her response as clearly as the long-ago day she said it.

"Because being older is unfair. That's how it is." End of discussion.

My mother was the oldest of four sisters. While I knew them, we weren't really close. My mother never shared any details of their youthful interactions, and I realize now that she carried childhood baggage of her own. I must have realized this to a degree even then, for I never broached the subject ever again.

When I turned nineteen, I decided I wanted a driver's license. Mother shut this down. Driving is risky, she said. No. Period. But I was older and craftier now. I devised a plan.

Every January, there is a national holiday known as Coming of Age Day. It celebrates citizens who turn twenty that year. Traditionally, when a woman turns twenty, her mother buys her a gorgeous long-sleeved kimono called a furisode. Municipalities host elaborate ceremonies where freshly minted adults are lauded and given certificates. Friends dress up in their finest and celebrate at parties afterward. The girls almost inevitably wear their furisode. Maybe it's a little analogous to the idea of prom at an American high school, though it takes place a few years later and isn't about finding a date.

Furisode are not cheap. They cost the equivalent of about $6,000. This just so happened to roughly coincide with the cost of attending a driving school. (It is notoriously expensive to get a license in Japan.) Don't buy me a kimono, I told my mother. Give me the money for driving school instead. She took the deal, and I got my driver's license. I didn't bother going to my city's coming-of-age ceremony, nor did I go to any parties. It somehow didn't feel right, after the bargain.

Two years later, when my sister turned twenty, my mother bought her a furisode, *and* sent her to driving school. On Coming of Age Day, mother sent her to a salon to fix her hair in a beautiful traditional style, then accompanied her to a local studio for photos. Of course, my sister attended the ceremony with her friends in tow and had a grand time. My mother took great vicarious pleasure in all this; she even borrowed another kimono from a neighbor for another round of photos later. She compiled them into an album that she showed off proudly to anyone who visited. Few noticed that only one of her daughters was pictured in it.

Shortly thereafter, my mother began suffering the first symptoms of her long illness and needed to be taken to a hospital for a more thorough examination than the local practitioner could give. My sister was still too inexperienced to be comfortable driving alone, and my father was too busy with work. So I took her.

"I'm so glad that you got a driver's license," she said along the way. "Letting you get one was the right thing to do."

So why did you make me fight for it? I wanted to ask. But what was done was done. It was obvious she'd made her peace with our deal. So had I, but it would be many years before I realized at what cost. In an attempt to assuage the sense of loss I'd felt at missing my coming of age, at sharing this experience with family and friends, I'd convinced myself that I didn't look good in a kimono. No, even more—that I looked ugly in one. Kimonos weren't for me, ever.

That twisted logic was how I justified the deal with my mother. It was the rationalization that let me bury my sadness and frustration and move on with my life.

Now, I don't tell you this story because I think my mother was a monster. She wasn't. Or that I believe myself deserving of pity, or even sympathy, really. I tell it because I think this kind of thing is utterly normal. We all have seeds of frustration sown deep within us. Maybe they were planted by interactions with parents, or siblings, or friends, or coworkers. But those seeds are always there, and they can blossom into anger if we don't care for them properly.

....

KAMI KNOW ANGER, TOO. WHEN YOU THINK ABOUT IT, THIS makes sense. Kami are avatars of the natural world, and nature can most certainly get angry. On the morning of March 11, 2011, the waters of the Pacific coast of Japan were placid. But at 2:46 that afternoon, a massive earthquake churned them into a terrifying agent of destruction, transforming a life-giving sea into a ferocious, deadly tsunami. Earthquakes, in turn, are frightening things. But there are two sides to them, too. Without the volcanic activity that drives them, Japan would lack many of the things we love: the iconic Mount Fuji, or hot spring resorts, or the ash-nourished fields that produce our abundant rice. Within every powerful kami, it is said, coexist a nigitama, literally "peaceful spirit," and an aratama, literally "wild spirit." The difference between peaceful and wild isn't that of good and evil. It's inherent to the nature of the kami, just as it is to nature itself. I wonder if this is one of the fundamental differences between the way Japan and the West see the world.

The eighteenth-century religious philosopher Norinaga Motoori captured this quantum worldview when he wrote,

"A kami's behavior may appear malicious, but in the end analysis actually represents a fortunate thing. So too may things people interpret as auspicious cloak ill fortune lurking beneath."

The Japanese in the olden days knew this, and they developed all sorts of ways of dealing with the fury of angry kami. One of these furies was something with which anyone who lived in the 2020s can sympathize.

"It was I who wrought the plague," declared Omononushi-no-kami to Emperor Sujin in the first century BCE, as recorded in the ancient *Kojiki*. "Venerate me. The curse will be lifted, and the people be safe once again." This sounds almost like a shakedown, but Omononushi wasn't a villain. He is one of the most powerful kami; in fact, his name is written with characters meaning "Master of Great Things." I don't see his demand as a form of intimidation but rather a message to us about the "angry" forces of the world, beyond human control. He was the very first to reveal this side of the kami to us, and the first to suggest how this anger might be appeased.

When the anger of kami is ignored or unacknowledged, they can unleash it on humans in what is known as a tatari—a curse of misfortune. There are many stories of kami growing angry in the *Kojiki*, but the most famous examples were actually once human. If someone of a certain social stature was willfully mistreated, dishonored, and killed, they might return from the grave with a literal vengeance. These expressions of human anger turned kami are called onryo—literally, angry ghosts, and their influence was once believed to be the source of all sorts of unpleasantness, from fatal lightning strikes to mass calamities such as floods, droughts, plagues, and earthquakes.

As a Tokyoite, I live with one of the angriest kami of

them all. His name is Masakado, and long ago he was human like us. He was a warrior, a samurai, who in the year 940 CE led his clan in a failed coup d'état against the emperor. His mortal life ended with his head on a pike. But his reputation only continued to grow. Over the centuries he emerged as one of the most feared figures in the entire pantheon of kami, and an invincible protector of the city in which I was born and raised.

It might seem odd that the loser of a rebellion—and one against the imperial family, no less!—be celebrated in Japan's capital. But Japanese folklore is filled with romanticized sagas of those who died in quest of unrealized goals. There's even an idiom describing this philosophy: "Hangan-bi'iki," which the historian Ivan Morris evocatively translated as "the nobility of failure" in a book of the same title. We feel some empathy for tragic heroes, even if we don't sympathize with their goals. We admire the force that drove them, a respect for the power of motivation and commitment and courage in the face of overwhelming odds.

Masakado was born into nobility, over a thousand years ago, but emerged as a hero of the people. Times were tough back then in the east of Japan, hinterlands far from the civilization of the capital in the west, Kyoto. Local magistrates squeezed their subjects for outrageously high taxes. A spate of natural disasters like floods and droughts heaped even more misery on the suffering populace. Eventually, enough was enough. Starving farmers began taking up arms against the officials who oppressed them.

Masakado lived on what now corresponds to the Boso Peninsula, adjacent to Tokyo. He became enmeshed in a dispute with his uncle, a local warlord who administrated the region by imperial decree. Some tales say the two bickered over a woman; others, over property. A series of minor skirmishes between supporters of both sides inflamed the conflict into a localized civil war. Eventually, Masakado got the upper hand, seizing control of the entire region.

Then he grew even more bold. He and his troops captured local imperial headquarters one after the other, to the delight of the starving masses, who relished seeing their tormentors' comeuppance. They cheered Masakado, and he in turn was buoyed by their passions. "Heaven has granted me a great fighting skill," he wrote in a missive. "Who among my peers can be compared with me?"

Masakado rode this wave of local sentiment to declare himself the New Emperor of the East. As you might imagine, this didn't sit well with the "old" emperor. In a series of battles over the next two months, Masakado scored victory after victory against imperial forces, edging ever closer to a final push into the capital in Kyoto. A 940 CE war chronicle paints the scene in epic terms:

> *Mounted on chargers like dragons, Masakado's warriors lead followers as numerous as the clouds. They brandish their whips and their horses' hooves resound; they are ready to cross a mountain range ten thousand miles long. Their hearts are high, their spirits are raised by their victory, and they are ready to vanquish an army of one hundred thousand warriors.*

But it was not to be. In the final conflict, Masakado's extended family joined forces with imperial soldiers to corner the rebel. Still Masakado refused to surrender. He fought to the last, until he was finally felled by "a heaven-sent arrow" (as the victors who wrote history saw it). So it was that Masakado perished alongside hundreds of his closest followers. The rebellion was over. But even after he died in battle, his courage and stubborn refusal to yield moved a great many people on both sides of the conflict.

As was custom of the time, imperial troops carried Masakado's severed head back to Kyoto for inspection by the emperor, who ordered it displayed on the Kamogawa riverbank as a message to any who might still have fight in them. Today this area roughly corresponds to Kyoto's Pontocho, an entertainment district filled with bustling izakaya whose balconies overlook the placid waters of the river. But in 940 CE, it was an execution ground, a gruesome and haunted place. So far as anyone expected, this would be Masakado's final resting spot. The public display of his head, the first recorded in Japanese history, was an extreme measure, a testament to the rage boiling on both sides of the conflict. "Since creation the court has seen many rebellions, but none that compare to this," fumed an imperial edict. "Now and again there have been those who yearn with treasonous spirit, but such meet always with the calamity of obliteration!"

Masakado may have been obliterated in life, but death proved another matter. The tales say his severed head atop the pike sparked to life. Its eyes opened wide and its mouth roared in anger, over and over again: "I shall find my body and battle once again!" Terrified authorities dithered for days over what to do. Suddenly, Masakado's head lifted off the pike and took flight, screaming off to the east in search of his body. It flew for quite a long distance, over the mountains and far to the east, before finally crashing to the earth. Locals who happened upon the head washed it in the waters of a pond as a sign of respect, then buried it. They called the spot Masakado-no-kubizuka, the Mound of Masakado's

Head. For a long time, it was a forlorn place on the out-skirts of an obscure fishing village named Edo. Today it sits in the very heart of Tokyo.

....

I'VE BEEN VISITING THE MOUND OF MASAKADO'S HEAD, ON and off, for twenty years. At first, I was motivated by mor-bid curiosity. I was the kind of girl who'd scour the library shelves for books about haunted spots, and even after I grew up, I'd find myself idly typing key words like *terrifying*, *frightening*, and *haunted* into search engines. And Masaka-do's head inevitably popped up. A thousand-year-old grave in the middle of the city—who wouldn't be intrigued? And really, how spooky could something surrounded by sky-scrapers be? That discrepancy between old and new, ancient and high-tech, stone and steel, made it feel all the more vis-ceral somehow.

Masakado's head rests in one of Japan's most expensive neighborhoods: Otemachi, a hub of finance, industry, and politics, the kind of place high-powered bankers and lobby-ists and consultants have their offices. His grave is a ten-minute walk from Tokyo Station, an intercity rail hub where more than four thousand trains and half a million travelers pass daily. The labyrinth of corridors and shopping arcades beneath the station is legendarily complicated. I've lived here almost my entire life and still get lost in them. When you walk here, especially at peak times, you're prac-tically carried along by a human tide of tourists, office workers, and students, through hallways lined with stalls and shops hawking every kind of food, service, and product imaginable. It's hard to believe that anything old might re-main around here, let alone something haunted.

The first time I visited the site was years ago, on a bright and sunny day, but chilly gusts channeled through the sky-scraper canyons that define the landscape in this part of town. As I pushed through the bluster, I got lost a few times, which shouldn't be surprising. I was looking for a patch of ground in the midst of a maze of buildings large enough to blot out the sky.

Finally, I found it: five stone stairsteps, right off the side-walk in an otherwise unremarkable city block. They led up to a little patch of trees and shrubbery, shadowed on three sides by tall office buildings. This was the mound.

At one edge stood a pair of stone monuments, flanked by square stone vases for flowers, with a dish for burning in-cense between them: a Buddhist-style grave. The monu-ments stood at roughly the height of an adult. One was a weather-beaten stone lantern said to be from the pond where Masakado's head was first washed. The other was an obelisk hewn from dark stone, inscribed deeply with char-acters reading "Namu Amibda Butsu" (Merciful Buddha) and "Lotus Amitabha." This was a posthumous Buddhist name bestowed upon Masakado in 1307, centuries after his death. The occasion for giving it to him was a tatari curse: an epidemic of plague gripped the region, and locals be-lieved Masakado's anger was fueling it. And so a temple held a ceremony intended to quell his anger. The marker I was looking at was a "new" one that had replaced the original a century ago.

Anywhere else—the countryside, a cemetery—this would have been an inconspicuous scene. Here, however, in the heart of the financial district, it all felt jarringly out of place. For a space surrounded by glass and steel and concrete, the atmosphere was strangely cave-like and damp from being enshrouded in the eternal shadow of skyscrapers. A tradi-tional Japanese-style wall of plaster topped by clay roof tiles bordered the site, its base scalloped by stunted shrubbery, the only green in the immediate vicinity.

This was a strange confluence of modernity and antiquity, but it didn't feel haunted to me. It felt like another dimension, a secret space lurking just outside our mundane realities. I could understand why it unsettled people, but I liked this place. Or perhaps it spoke to me? Whatever the case, Masakado had some seriously high-powered neighbors. The rest of the block was filled with towers bearing big corporate names like Mitsubishi and the Four Seasons—and then at the end of the street stood the emperor's moat and palace. On any other block in this part of town, this plot would have been occupied by a skyscraper, too. But it sat empty save the grave.

In March 2020, the plot on which Masakado's grave sits was estimated to be worth a little over four billion yen: about thirty-five million US dollars. As you might expect, more than a few people have made a play for this juicy piece of real estate over the decades. But each and every time, something terrible happens to them. In 1924, the Ministry of the Treasury razed the mound to expand their offices. As they prepared to put up a prefab building on the site, the minister of the treasury died. Then the construction foreman died. Over the next few weeks, another twelve bureaucrats in the ministry died. This so spooked the government that they hastily re-erected the monument and organized a chinkonsai. This is a Shinto ceremony sometimes translated as an "exorcism" but more specifically is a memorial ritual intended to soothe disturbed souls, whether human or kami, so they may rest. This might have been superstition, but it was also major news. SPIRIT OF MASAKADO! WE APOLOGIZE! read one paper's headline, with the subtitle TERRIFIED GOVERNMENT MINISTERS HOLD A CHINKONSAI. It worked for a while, but then, in 1940, a bolt of lightning struck the Ministry of the Treasury, sparking a blaze that reduced the entire block to ashes. The government performed another memorial ritual.

In 1946, just after the war, history repeated. The Allied forces now occupied the area. Someone decided that they wanted to turn Masakado's plot into a parking lot, and sent in a military bulldozer to flatten the mound. But things again went terribly wrong. The machine flipped over for some reason, killing its driver. Japanese officials convinced the Americans to abandon the plan.

The governments of two mighty nations tried and failed to move this plot of earth. That's what makes Masakado so endlessly fascinating. He was in many ways the prototypical samurai, a warrior who literally died in his saddle; and he continues to manifest his fury today, resolutely unfazed by what we consider our more advanced civilization.

In Japanese idiom, anger is linked to three parts of the body: the belly, the chest, and the head. Traditionally, the belly is believed to be the repository of all emotions. When we want to have a frank discussion, we don't have a heart-to-heart; we "hara wo watte hanasu"—"crack open our stomachs." So long as anger dwells in the stomach, it can be contained, hidden. When for whatever reason it can't be, anger rises to the chest and agitates us. And should something then push us over the edge, it rises to our heads and we explode in visible anger. We have a word for anger, *ikari*, but it sounds more poetic than visceral. In actual conversation, the way someone is most likely to express how angry they feel is through the phrase "atama ni kita," which literally means "it came to my head." Is this why we find the story of Masakado's furious head taking on a life of its own so compelling? It certainly fits.

The longer we live, the more life experiences we accumulate. But the journey isn't always smooth. There will inevitably be uncomfortable patches, too. Hopefully, our lives, on balance, will be happy and satisfying ones. But the older we grow, the more negative things we will naturally experience. Some of these are slights we can brush off; others cut deeper, sticking with us, forming a pool of negative energy within us. It bubbles deep in our minds like magma, inexorably seeking fissures caused by stress, frustration, or even errant memories. Then it seeps out—or it erupts.

LIKE MANY PEOPLE TRAPPED INDOORS DURING THE EARLY months of the COVID-19 pandemic, I cast around for ways to occupy my time. A few months before the outbreak sent us all indoors, I had inherited a piece of furniture from my great-aunt, a beautiful old chest made of paulownia wood, light but strong. It stood about the height of my head, and each of its deep drawers was filled with her old kimonos. They were in beautiful condition. Nobody else in the family, close or extended, expressed any interest in keeping them. And so they found their way to me.

I had no experience wearing a kimono myself, but I couldn't bear to see my great-aunt's treasures tossed out or given away. And I was fascinated by their age, their tradition, their craft. Plus, I was about to turn fifty. Why not learn a few new tricks? Japan is home to many kimono schools; they help keep the old traditions alive in our modern era, even as most have fully embraced Western fashions. I enrolled in a local class. It consisted of weekly workshops whose logistics were made complex by viral countermeasures. We had to work in a room whose windows were thrown wide open regardless of how frigid or muggy it was outside, and when the time came to practice putting a kimono on someone else, we had to use mannequins instead of one another, to maintain social distance. The curriculum would last a year and a half, and at the end of it, we would be certified as licensed kimono fitters—the first step in becoming teachers ourselves, if we so desired. I didn't have any aspirations of hanging out my shingle; I simply wanted to learn the basics of the traditional art of dressing up, and this was the best way to do it.

There are many types of kimono, made of different materials, and there are precise rules for who can wear each of them and at which times. This complexity is exactly what scares many modern Japanese away from wearing them, but I found myself fascinated by the intricacies of it all. Our teacher was a petite woman in her sixties who was a retired kindergarten teacher, and meticulously instructed us in gentle tones borne of years wrangling far more rambunctious students than us. She taught how to wear each type of kimono in turn, even types we wouldn't normally wear, including hakama, which are kimono for men. Inevitably, the day came when we began learning about furisode.

Furisode are intended for unmarried young women to wear during celebrations, which is why they're de rigueur for Coming of Age Day. They're strikingly colorful and meticulously embroidered with auspicious designs such as flowers or birds. And they're instantly recognizable from their oversize sleeves, the bottom edges of which dangle almost to the ground. Even though we were all middle-aged women, as licensed fitters we might very well have to help some youngster prepare for her coming of age one day. To be honest, I didn't think much about the implications of this on the day of class, for I was too busy following the teacher's instructions, immersed in the trickiness of putting a kimono on a mannequin, a task I'd only barely mastered on myself.

It wasn't until the next morning that it hit me. When I was brushing my teeth, of course.

All the memories of my bargain with my mother came rushing back in a cascade of connected flashes. Mental movies of battles waged between the two of us, playing out in fast-forward as I groggily looked at myself in the mirror. And then came my old rationalizations, bubbling up from the depths of my unconscious.

Kimonos aren't for me.

I don't even like kimonos.

I'll look ugly in a kimono.

Yeah, skipping the kimono was the right move.

How could I ever have convinced myself I'd look ugly in such a beautiful garment? It was a testament to how desperate I was to avoid feeling the pain of that long-ago deal. I'd created this new version of reality, in which the kimono and I could never meet, and planted it deep within my mind. Where it sat, unremembered, for decades. What obstinacy! Now, thirty years later, my mouth foaming with toothpaste, I found my anger rising. At my mother. At the situation. And most of all at myself.

AFTER MY MOTHER'S DEATH, I FOUND MYSELF DRAWN TO Masakado's story again. I visited the mound whenever I happened to be in that section of town, and discovered that there was another spot dedicated to his memory in the city: Kanda Shrine, located near Ochanomizu Station. The mound was a grave, but Kanda Shrine venerated Masakado officially, a man's memory turned kami. There I learned of a network of smaller shrines dedicated to him as well.

Masakado is famed as an icon of anger, a sleeping tiger who occasionally awakens with a roar. Those roars literally shook the city over the centuries, in the form of earthquakes and other calamities attributed to his fury. Yet the people love him dearly nonetheless. How could a god of anger be the object of so much love? Respect I could understand, but this went beyond that. And our appreciation of Masakado extends from the streets of the city to the heavens—not metaphorically but literally.

Even in modern Tokyo's bright skies, where the shine of countless streetlamps and signboards and office towers means true darkness never quite falls, the Big Dipper is visible glimmering in the heavens above. The pattern is mirrored in the city below, in a series of holy spots whose positions were carefully chosen to mimic the shape of the constellation when viewed on a map. One of them is the mound of Masakado's head. Another is Kanda Shrine. And the rest, that network of smaller shrines I learned about, venerate Masakado, too. This didn't happen by chance. They were arranged this way many centuries ago at the order of a man named Tokugawa Ieyasu—then-shogun of Japan, ruler of all the land.

Ieyasu came of age during a period so tumultuous it is now known as the Era of Warring States. He would eventually end this strife by surviving many intrigues and winning many battles. Along the way, Ieyasu turned to the kami for assistance. He prayed often at Kanda Shrine for victory on the battlefield. His greatest triumph came in 1600 at the epic Battle of Sekigahara. Total victory allowed him to unify all of Japan under his control. Afterward, he bestowed great riches upon Kanda Shrine in appreciation. Ieyasu's patronage elevated the shrine, and Masakado, from a local curiosity into the protector of the entire city.

And then he took a bold step. Under the advice of his spiritual adviser, a Buddhist monk, Ieyasu relocated Kanda Shrine, along with a series of other, smaller shrines dedicated to Masakado, so that they would form the shape of the Big Dipper. The mound of Masakado's head, the only one to stay in place, formed the bottom corner of the dipper's cup.

Certain schools of Buddhism had long venerated the constellation, but now Ieyasu assumed it as his personal emblem, a symbol of his authority that would shine over his people forever. Stitching Masakado's shrines together into the pattern was a show of respect by association, but it was also a form of sorcery, a magical barrier intended to pacify Masakado and keep the city safe from his wrath. One might read into it something else: a message to potential rivals. The political subtext of a shogun venerating Masakado, who fought imperial authority to his dying breath, must have been abundantly clear to the emperor, now cloistered in Kyoto.

The shogun is long gone; Ieyasu died in 1616. But the Big Dipper remains in the heavens above and etched into the streets of the city below. In the city where I live. Not many realize that a magical spell is woven into Tokyo's map, but it's true, and it's a spell designed around anger. Most would see this as a quaint artifact of ancient history. But I was starting to wonder if it might still be relevant, with a bigger message about dealing with anger: how to recognize it, channel it, and even cultivate it for more productive uses.

I told myself that the furisode module would be over soon, and I could go back to forgetting about my youthful anger. But as it turned out, that wouldn't be possible.

With the help of our instructor, the seven of us passed our practical and written exams. We were now licensed kimono fitters, armed with the know-how to dress ourselves, or advise others, in traditional fashions.

Mastering the basics, as we had, was a pretty fancy skill to have. But still, they were only the basics. For instance, the obi belts. We had only mastered the most common form of fastening them, known as the drum knot. It was the proper choice for the vast majority of situations. But for those so inclined, there are many other ways of tying an obi, each with its own evocative name: the wisteria, the chrysanthemum, the leaves of bamboo, just to name a few. So even with our certifications, there was more to learn. Buoyed by the shared camaraderie of having passed our studies during a difficult time, plus simply enjoying one another's company, we made a group decision to push ahead to the next level.

The curriculum would consist of a mixture of lectures, field trips to kimono workshops and factories all over Japan, and classroom practice, just as it had for our basic certification. But there was a twist. This semester would focus almost entirely on the furisode.

To say this stirred complicated feelings in me would be an understatement. Having to deal with the thing in my previous course had been unsettling enough. Now I would have to face it every class. It felt like a sleeping tiger had been awakened, pacing within the confines of my mind. Again the dark thoughts began to emerge as I brushed my teeth in the mornings.

Yet it never occurred to me to quit. My sensei was a great instructor, and for this course was joined by a second, a cheerful mother of three from the Kansai region. The other students were more than just attentive learners; we'd become friends. And I knew that the studying of new things always energized me. So I forged on.

Still, it stung every time I interacted with a furisode.

During sensei's lecture, or during hands-on practice, even while simply looking at one folded up—a bitterness arose in me, unbidden from deep within. I resolved to double down on my studies, but the mind naturally wanders, and whenever it did, I found myself slipping into a past I'd tried desperately to escape.

One moment I was here; the next I'd be nineteen years old, in the kitchen, having that argument with my mother. It was as though I was pulled back in time, over and over. Arguing, over and over. Angry, over and over. I'd wrest myself back into the present, will myself to forget about the past, to keep it dead and buried. This never worked. So it was that I found myself caught up in a cursed dance with the furisode, and it continued for the better part of a year.

My instinct was to exorcize this anger somehow, banish it so it would cease to trouble me. But the more I visited Masakado's head, that star in the constellation stretching across Tokyo, the more I started to think: Maybe my anger isn't ever going away. And maybe it doesn't have to. We never forgot Masakado's anger. It keeps roaring back from time to time to remind us of his existence.

When the Tokugawa Shogunate fell and Emperor Meiji reasserted control over Japan in 1868, he launched an ambitious and controversial modernization program called the Meiji Restoration. Once again, it put Masakado, or rather the memory of him, at loggerheads with the imperial family.

With the shogun out and the emperor back in charge, Masakado was seen as a traitor once again. Given that he'd been dead for almost a thousand years by this point, you might imagine this a conceptual formality. But it had very real impacts on daily life. When the Emperor Meiji paid a visit to Kanda Shrine, the priests "demoted" Masakado from the main shrine into a lesser shrine on the grounds. Their aim was to avoid causing offense, but the move infuriated local parishioners.

The imperial government's modernization plan meant developing infrastructure. When the time came to build the Yamanote Line, the train loop that encircles Tokyo, the tracks needed to intersect the "lines" of the Big Dipper constellation in two spots. The final section of rail, which intersected the line between Masakado's head mound and another shrine venerating his samurai helm, was due to be completed in 1923. But just before the final track could be laid, the Great Kanto Earthquake leveled the city. More than a hundred thousand people lost their lives that day.

A curse? Coincidence? Urban legend? Perhaps. But the damage suffered by the treasury and later the US Armed Forces in their interactions with Masakado's mound cemented his reputation all the more. Years of public pressure led Kanda Shrine to reverse course and reenshrine Masakado in 1984. A thousand citizens, many dressed in Edo Era fashions, attended the ceremony to cheer him on. Now, every odd-numbered year, the shrine hosts one of Japan's biggest festivals, parading a float dedicated to Masakado through the streets of the city, thronged by a crowd that often reaches a hundred thousand strong.

In 2021, the Mound of Masakado's Head underwent a major renovation. Gone are the trees and shadows, concrete walls and even soil; now it is an airy open space surrounded by latticework fencing built from lengths of metal and glass. Crushed stone crunches underfoot as you approach the monuments, the only vestiges of the former site: that century-old pillar and far older stone lantern. I'm not sure how I feel about this makeover, to be honest. It's very fancy, to be sure; very stark, very modern, even chic. I think I preferred the intimacy of the original space, with its damp and organic feel, like a thousand years of history hiding in plain sight. But change isn't necessarily a bad thing, either. It shows how much care we lavish on Masakado even today.

The Ministry of the Treasury, which suffered so much of Masakado's wrath over the years, is now known as the Ministry of Finance. It hosts a detailed report of Masakado's life and history on its website. The skyscrapers surrounding the Mound of Masakado's Head have been carefully designed so that their windows do not loom over the spot; if you look carefully, you can see offsets in the facades of the buildings around the site, artfully crafted so as to give Masakado a respectful amount of "breathing room." Local businesses pool their money to pay for daily cleanings, regular maintenance, and annual ritual ceremonies. This is all managed through the local branch of Japan's biggest bank, which collects the donations not only from the firms but from visitors to the mound who leave offerings. The funds are all held under the name Taira Masakado, making him the only kami, angry or otherwise, to possess a bank account.

Masakado is angry and the people love him for it. That's because he isn't angry *at* us; he's angry *for* us. His anger is part of what makes him *him*, and in turn all of us *us*.

Could the same be true on a personal level? Maybe I could love my mother and myself in spite of the anger that so often defined our interactions, and now dominated my memories. Maybe anger wasn't a sign of failure but rather part of our shared identity.

....

ONE DAY, A THOUGHT LEAPT INTO MY MIND, AS UNBIDDEN as the usual flashes of negativity. But this time, it was different.

Wow. I'm really hurting. All those fights really hurt me.

This might sound like a no-brainer to you, after reading all this, but sometimes the closest truths are the most difficult to see. The words felt as though they were being spoken to me by someone else. I'd buried that hurt under anger for so long, I'd forgotten I was even hurt in the first place, as though I'd mistaken scar tissue for skin. The more I looked, metaphorically speaking, the more shocked I was at the lumps I'd taken, and that I continued to give myself. This sparked a new feeling within: pity. Not for me, not the me of now, but for the younger me, the teenager who still seemed to dwell deep inside.

When I looked at this place where I had buried my feelings, I realized there was a great sadness underneath. It was as though digging beneath the surface released voices from within, which swirled and dipped around me like a whirlwind.

I wish she'd bought me a furisode. I wish I could have celebrated my coming of age in it, just like everyone else. Just like my sister.

Fortunately, this never affected my relationship with my sister. We were and are best friends, always looking after each other. But it's a fact that whenever my mother said her name in comparison with mine, it triggered simmering fury. I'd recognized this, and once even tried calling my mother out on her favoritism. But the swiftness with which she shut that conversation down made things worse. She'd considered the conversation over. I suspect she didn't even remember it. And looking back at it with the benefit of many years of hindsight, I don't even think she meant offense. But I never forgot. To me, the conversation wasn't over at all. Now my mother was gone, and there was no way to finish it. The only thing that remained was anger and frustration. I'd buried it like one might smother embers with earth, but they kept smoldering, until the contact with the furisode caused them to burst into flame once again.

But I knew it wasn't really about the kimono at all. It was about me, and my mother. That actually made it worse, because she was dead. You'd think the end of a strained relationship would bring closure, but it doesn't. The strain amplifies the loss all the more. I was mourning a person, but also an idea, an ideal, of how it could have been. The living can never win an argument with the dead, for the dead always have the last word. Unresolved issues: Maybe that's what a haunting really is.

Even now, nearly twenty years after she'd departed the world of the living, I still saw myself orbiting her, like some dark star. But the time had come for me to break away.

And slowly, things started changing. The kimono school provided a great many different types of kimono and obi for practice, all of them gorgeous. Every class began with students picking one they liked, then pairing it with one of the many accessories the school stocked for that purpose: things like obijime, the cords used to keep obi in place, or obiage, scarf-like pieces of fabric that can be used to add more color to an outfit. Under the watchful eye of our sensei, we practiced fitting them to mannequins over and over, our goal singular: *Make it look pretty.* At first I had struggled to make my furisode look good, or rather, to see it as looking good. But now I began to reframe my efforts. The mannequin I was dressing wasn't an opponent but an avatar: me, many years ago, when I was still a teen. "Big me" began talking to "teenage me," filling in the blanks where the hole of my mother had been, and always would be. *Which furisode would you like to wear today? Which obi?*

Toward the end of the semester, our teachers announced that there'd be a little competition on the very last day of class. The rules were simple: Each of us was to dress a mannequin in a furisode, and complete the outfit with an obi tied in a totally original way—none of the classics, but something each of us thought up ourselves. Then we'd all score one another on style and technique, and the highest would be declared the winner. This wasn't a battle; it wouldn't affect our passing the course, and there wasn't any prize other than the winner getting their mannequin displayed in the entryway of the school for a few weeks. It was simply a fun way to celebrate the things we'd learned together. Still, we all took it seriously and began practicing in class for the month leading up to the big event.

The day of the competition happened to fall at the end of the Year of the Rabbit, so I picked a furisode with a fun motif suiting the season. It featured sprays of pastel flowers against a black background. If you looked closely, you could spot white bunnies, so artfully incorporated into the design you might miss them at first glance, leaping though the blossoms as though frolicking in snow. It was a perfect balance between beauty and cute factor, a combination that reminded me of the threshold between youth and adulthood.

I took special care in fitting the furisode to the mannequin. The art of the kimono is measured in folds so subtle they might seem imperceptible to outsiders, but to those in the know, even the tiniest of adjustments can make a big difference. Varying the dip of the collar so as to cover or expose the nape of the neck, or the fold of the lapels by an inch or less, can mean the difference between looking older or younger, naive or flirtatious. So I made sure to fit the furisode in a way that telegraphed the confidence of the young woman I imagined was wearing it.

Next I took an obi, white fabric embroidered with silver thread that glinted under the lights, and carefully began to wrap and fold it. In the two years since I'd started the course, I'd learned many ways to tie an obi. But this would be the first time I'd be making my own design for public viewing. I took my time, spending a half hour getting the material into the curves I'd worked out in practice sessions. When it comes to kimono, a tiny mismatch or misfold early on can carry through like ripples in a pond, amplifying any lapses and diminishing the appearance of the final result.

My design was based on the drum knot, that elegant rounded knot that sits in the center of the woman's back. But I folded it in a more complex geometry that resulted in pair of "wings" angling up from the knot in back, as though the entire arrangement were about to take flight. I called it ogi-cho—the fan-butterfly. I saw it as a gift from myself to the me of the past, a retroactive celebration of that coming of age I'd missed so long ago. A present only I could give myself.

Afterward, we toured the room and oohed and aahed over one another's designs. I was impressed by the work of my fellow students, each of whom, like me, had incorporated their own themes and personalities into the fitting of their kimono. Then the time came for the teachers to announce the scores. They were very close, they told us; we'd all shown just how far we'd come. But one scored just a little higher than the rest.

Mine.

I couldn't believe it. It wasn't that I thought I hadn't done a good job but rather that I was surrounded by talent. And winning didn't feel like a triumph so much as a celebration— all of us had studied so hard, and this was the culmination of all that effort and work. It didn't feel like a personal victory, but a shared one. Not only among my fellow students, but within myself, of now-me and then-me.

My furisode with its sash tied in its butterfly design stood in the front lobby of the school for two weeks, and my teachers later said that it had gotten a lot of praise whenever people came for events. That made me very happy, of course. But proud as I was to see my handiwork recognized, I was happier still that I'd made my peace with the furisode. And my mother. Was that butterfly a symbol of the metamorphosis of my feelings toward her? Honestly, it hadn't been on my mind, not consciously, when I first began planning out what kind of obi knot I'd make. It was a strange thing.

I still get angry about the past from time to time. But I've stopped trying to bury those feelings. When the memories come flooding back, I can admit how upset or disappointed or sad I was back then, which is to say I respect those feelings. This acceptance is a tool for bringing the anger back under control. In a way, it's as though I built my own "mound" in my mind, a place I can visit from time to time without getting overwhelmed. I've come to realize that those feelings of anger are part of me, part of the energies swirling within that motivated me to go to kimono classes week after week, month after month, even after I'd long ago convinced myself I looked ugly in a kimono.

These days, I make a habit of wearing a kimono out, once or twice a week. It isn't nearly as common to see women in a kimono on the streets as it once was, and I'm always surprised at how many compliments I get from strangers, young and old. I've come to think of these voices out of the blue as the kami speaking to me, watching over me and telling me everything's going to be all right.

CHAPTER 5

Belief without Belief: Hanshin-Hangi

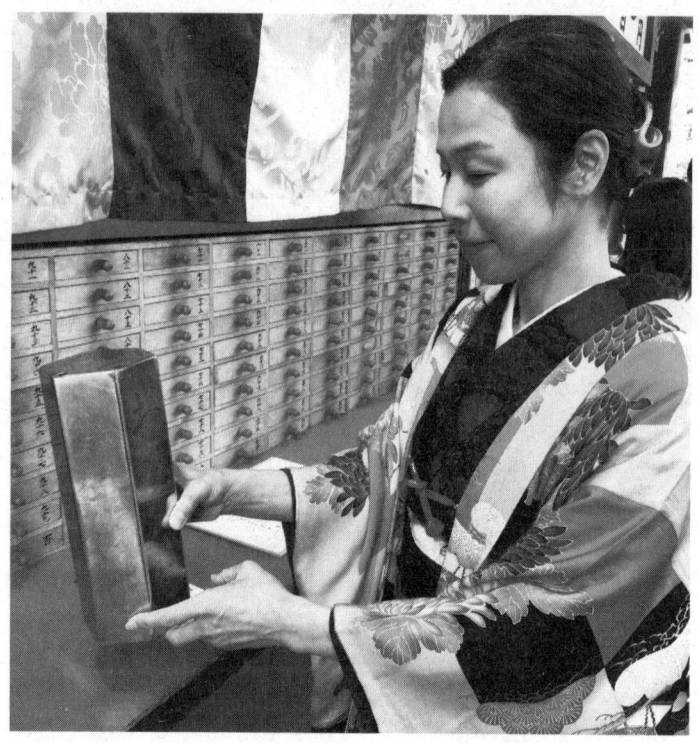

Reading my fortune at Sensoji temple in Tokyo.

Respect the kami and Buddhas, but do not depend on them.

—Miyamoto Musashi

Almost 70 percent of Japanese claim not to believe in fortune-telling. I am one of them. Yet when many Japanese visit temples and shrines, they get their fortunes told. I am one of *them*, too. And I am not in the minority. According to surveys, more than half of those who ring in the New Year at a temple or shrine also get their fortunes read along the way. How to explain this seeming paradox?

I believe I am the master of my own fate. But I don't believe I am in total control, either. Life is complicated and chaotic. There are so many ways in which the best-laid plans can go awry, often for reasons impossible to predict. But humans are hardwired to believe in cause and effect. This is where a desire to know one's fortune enters the picture. It's kind of like a road map for your future, as believers see it. But what some call fate, I prefer to think of as "kami territory."

"God does play dice with the universe," wrote the physicist Stephen Hawking. "All the evidence points to him being an inveterate gambler, who throws the dice on every possible occasion." When Hawking says "God," he isn't speaking of religious deities but nature itself, which in quantum mechanics exists in probabilities rather than absolutes. That's how I mean "kami" in this context, too. Not in a literal sense but as a shorthand for the unknowable and the unpredictable. To me, kami territory is where those metaphorical dice are thrown.

Given the unknowability of the, well, unknowable, I am very leery of anyone who claims a direct line to the fates, or God, kami, Buddha, or whatever higher power. On the occasions I feel like getting a fortune, I prefer to get it myself. Fortunately, over many generations, Japanese have developed all sorts of tools for self-diagnosing one's fate. The most popular of these is called omikuji, the drawing of sacred lots, in which you vigorously shake a cylinder filled with rods until one pops out of a tiny hole in the top. Many temples and shrines offer this service to visitors for a small fee. Even if you don't take the outcome seriously, it can be fun to do, which is why I see so many people, natives and tourists alike, reading their fortunes this way at holy spots in Japan.

I'm not a genius like Hawking. I don't know quantum mechanics, but I do know *hanshin-hangi*—a Japanese idiom that means "half belief, half disbelief." It's a kind of quantum state of mind. In English, belief and disbelief lie at opposite ends of a spectrum. Normally, they do so in Japanese as well. But hanshin-hangi contextualizes belief and disbelief differently, as complements rather than rivals. In our cultural traditions, belief and disbelief don't have to oppose. In fact, they can be mutually *inclusive*, comfortably sitting side by side in one's mind. As a result, the question of whether one believes something has far more flexibility.

The English phrase "cognitive dissonance" describes the mental stress one feels when confronted by contradictory pieces of information. But "hanshin-hangi" isn't an expression of stress. It's the opposite: embracing paradox so as to let contradictions coexist side by side. Let me be clear: This isn't some kind of far-out New Age philosophy. It isn't rooted in any religious doctrine or faith. It's simply a mindset, a mental tool for handling the paradoxes life throws at us.

Think of it like one of those old analog sound volume dials, but applied instead to concepts: a "belief meter," where the balance between two or even more conflicting ideas can be adjusted as needed, case by case, based on instinct, emotion, or knowledge, to arrive at a comfortable equilibrium. It reconciles conflicts by letting you have your cake and eat it, too. *Does Santa Claus exist? Logically, it makes no sense, but wouldn't it be nice if he did? Do fortunes come true? I don't know, but it's New Year's Day—why not see what this year has in store?*

I should emphasize here that hanshin-hangi is applicable only to things widely considered pretty harmless—a belief in ghosts, or fairies, or fortunes, or anything that can't really be proved one way or another but that doesn't cause much trouble one way or the other, either. If a belief does prove damaging or detrimental, that's a different story. There's a phrase I've heard in English: "You are entitled to own your opinion. But you are not entitled to your own facts." If facts are on the table, hanshin-hangi is out, and debate comes into play.

The ability to believe and disbelieve simultaneously isn't some mental game. It's a way of looking at the world that is rooted in respect—respect born from a recognition of the fact that there are many things beyond your power to control. Belief implies a personal agency that I (and I suspect many Japanese) feel is at odds with the great unknowables that the kami represent. If you were to ask me, *Do you believe in kami?*, I wouldn't know how to answer. What authority do I have to conjure them into existence, or to declare them nonexistent? What right? When you're talking about things as profound as the mysteries of the universe, which is really what kami are, declaring belief can feel a little presumptuous, even arrogant.

This isn't dodging the question. To me, respect trumps belief. I suspect even Hawking would have been the first to agree that gravity doesn't care if you believe in it. All that matters is your respect, as expressed through what you do—such as choosing not to walk off a cliff. My relationship with the kami is similar. It doesn't matter whether I believe, only what I do—in this case, showing my respect at a shrine, or wherever and however I feel it appropriate.

I feel that fortune-telling, or Japan's seemingly contradictory approach to it, functions like a lens into this worldview. How is it that I and so many of my fellow citizens do things we claim to disbelieve in? How is that seemingly contradictory thinking compatible with a modern life? And why do I find this worldview to be so important?

These are big questions. And I realize as I ask them that this duality, this pluralism, this ability to see and hold opposing ideas in mind at once, represents a kind of pulse echoing throughout my life, sometimes quiet, sometimes thundering. That pulse quickened the very first time I started thinking about the kami, sharpened through my adolescent explorations of spirituality, amplified through my interactions with foreigners, then reached a crescendo during the profound losses of my parents.

Looking back, it was from the kami that I picked up this pluralistic approach to spirituality, very early on. It wasn't some kind of religious teaching, or moral training. In fact, I don't think my parents were even aware they were teaching me hanshin-hangi themselves.

My mother was a pragmatic homemaker. My father was an entrepreneur. Neither seemed to believe in fortune-telling. I recall one time, when I was quite young, when my mother came back home in a huff from a tea party with friends.

"I'd never let a stranger tell us what they thought was wrong with *our* house," she fumed to father. I gathered that one of her friends had dominated the conversation with the results of a fortune-teller she had hired to analyze her home. "What can you do about a house that's already built?" she continued. "Even if there *was* something 'wrong' with our house, which there *isn't*, I wouldn't want to hear about it."

On the other hand, neither did my parents reject the concept of fortunes entirely. Another time, they went on a trip of some kind for a few days and left my sister and me in the care of our aunt and uncle. I remember it well, because it was like a vacation for us, too. My cousins were a rambunctious trio of brothers a few years older than us, who obligingly incorporated us into their wrestling matches and mock battles. My uncle would sometimes join in, tossing us playfully in the air. And when we grew overstimulated by the horseplay, we would take refuge with my aunt, who doted on us like the daughters she never had.

My parents returned bearing a present: an omamori. *Omamori* literally means "special protection." They are little amulets. You'll see them arranged in neat rows for sale at many temples and shrines—essentially, spiritual souvenirs. That both Shinto shrines and Buddhist temples sell these things is another example of how seamlessly various faith traditions coexist here in Japan. The details differ from place to place, but the underlying concept is basically the same: protecting against misfortunes, ushering in good luck. Some take the form of tiny cloth sacks with pretty patterns, soft containers for talismans within. Others are more like key chains, ranging from simple geometric shapes to flowers, figurines, bells, or even tiny frogs, whose Japanese name, kaeru, is a homonym for "returning safely."

Omamori aren't expensive. They're usually priced at under

a thousand yen, less than ten dollars, so anyone can buy them for a little metaphysical support whenever they need it. On a job search, say, or getting treatment for an illness, or studying for exams, or looking for love. Others are intended for longer-term protection. It isn't at all uncommon to keep an omamori inside a car to avoid traffic accidents, or to tie one to a child's backpack to keep them safe when commuting. I've even seen one that purports to protect against the loss of computer data.

Nobody believes an amulet is a substitute for common sense—even the staunchest believer in traffic omamori would never dare cross a busy street without looking both ways first. But these amulets are ubiquitous in Japan, and have been for as long as anyone can remember.

The most traditional are very simple: hand-printed talismans that are wrapped up in a crisp sheet of washi paper, which you are never supposed to open. The omamori my parents gave me was of this variety. I had no idea what it was. To my seven-year-old eyes it wasn't much of a souvenir. It was inscribed with kanji calligraphy, but I couldn't yet read it. And it looked like a letter, but I was told I wasn't allowed to open it. *Boring.* "This is an omamori, Hiroko," my mother said. "It's from the kami-sama, and it will protect you."

This was, I now realize, the first time I'd ever heard the word *kami*. I knew all about kaiju because that was what we called the monsters on TV shows like *Ultraman* or *Five Rangers*, big hits among the schoolyard set. I knew *obaké*, the Japanese word for spooks and ghosts, from that picture book I'd found in my classroom, *Little Obaké and Muwamuwa-mu*. But *kami* was a new one for me.

Protection was something I understood. The superheroes of my favorite shows would declare their mission to "keep the peace" and "fight for justice" before swooping in to save a school bus of kids from yet another dastardly kaiju. And I had the sense that these kami, whatever they were, must be pretty important, because my mother referred to them with the honorific -sama, which was even more polite than appending -san to someone's name. Put the pieces together and it was obvious: This was something worthy of respect.

I had a study desk, with a little bookshelf integrated into the back. I put the omamori on the top shelf, as high as I could. Writing it out like this, I am realizing that, already at this young age, and without any real prompting from my family, I was constructing a rudimentary kamidana altar.

Then I promptly forgot about it. This isn't surprising. An omamori wasn't something I could play with. At the end of the school year, six months or so later, my mother asked my sister and me to clean up our desks. She handed each of us a big plastic garbage bag and told us to fill them with anything we didn't want anymore.

I took this task seriously, examining each and every piece of paper, toy, pencil, origami animal, and figurine that had accrued in my workspace over the months. Did I need it? Did it spark joy, to borrow a modern turn of phrase? I started at the bottom of my desk, working through each drawer, then the desktop, keeping what I needed and discarding what I didn't. Finally, I reached the bookshelf at the very top.

And there it was, the talisman, now covered with a coat of dust. I picked it up and contemplated it for some time. I knew it was something special, somehow different from the other stuff I owned. It was a protector, I'd been told, connected to this mysterious kami-sama. And it had been a gift from my parents. On the other hand, let's be honest: It was basically a piece of paper. Had I noticed any particular special effects from having it in my possession? I couldn't think of any. *Still, I'd better keep it*, I thought. But just as suddenly, the cleaning prerogative took hold. *It's just an old piece of paper.* I dropped it into the garbage bag, and before long, it was buried in other detritus from my room. When I was done, I tied up the bag and handed it to my mother. I never mentioned the omamori.

And that was that.

Or so I thought. No sooner had I handed off the garbage than I began noticing something strange. The house was making creaking noises. They seemed particularly loud around my desk and in my bedroom. This wasn't the first time I'd heard the house making noises. Once, after hearing creaks at night, I'd asked my father what they meant. He'd explained that it was only the sound of the house settling under its own weight as the lumber dried out. That had satisfied me then, but now things felt different. It was during the day, loud, and all around me.

My sister and I shared two rooms. We slept in one and studied in the other. Despite the fact that we spent our days in close proximity, she didn't seem to register these sounds at all. When I asked, she just shrugged. For some reason this made me even more uneasy.

I couldn't get the omamori out of my mind. I'd sensed it was wrong to throw the talisman away, but I'd done this nonetheless. *Are the kami-sama mad at me?* I told myself it was all in my imagination. But the sounds didn't stop—or perhaps I simply couldn't stop noticing them. I grew scared. *They must be angry with me!*

My parents always said that when you wronged someone, you needed to make amends with a direct apology. That was just fundamental, commonsense courtesy. I began to feel as though I needed to apologize to the kami-sama. The only problem was, I'd never met them. I couldn't even see them. So I did the next best thing. I climbed on my bed to get as high as possible. I put my palms together, just like I'd seen family members do at my grandparents' grave, and gazed up to the ceiling. Then I said, "I'm sorry."

And with that, the sounds abruptly stopped. It seemed as though the kami-sama accepted my apology.

Now, don't get me wrong. I am not suggesting this was some kind of paranormal activity. This was no *Poltergeist*, to name-check a favorite movie of the era. I've always believed that these experiences were in my head, a reaction to and interpretation of what was happening around me in the moment. Still, I cherish this memory, partly out of childhood nostalgia, but mainly because it sparked an epiphany, even at that very young age. Even the most boring-looking sheet of paper might become something frighteningly powerful if you think about it in a certain way. But most of all, I treasure it as the moment my parents, who didn't seem to believe in fortunes at all, unwittingly introduced me to the concept of kami and that they were worthy of respect. A respect I could express in my own little-girl way.

MY INTRODUCTION TO FORTUNE-TELLING CAME SEVERAL years later, when I was old enough to start getting an allowance: a thousand yen a month in ten hundred-yen coins, the equivalent of a few dollars. When my parents began giving me this money, my mother told me I'd need a coin bank to keep it in. She took me to the local Sanrio shop—you may know that name, because it's the same company that created Hello Kitty. Their shops sold all sorts of things, from stationery to accessories, like a fashion boutique designed just for girls. Coin banks were among their merchandise. I chose one shaped like a little boy in robes, carrying a big yellow star on his back.

The bank was made of fragile ceramic. I loved the feel of its smooth, glazed surface against my skin, and its shape nestled eagerly in my hands, as though it wanted to be there.

The boy had a name, Kiki, and the story went that he was the younger brother of a girl named Lala. Together they were known as the Little Twin Stars—a personification of the Gemini twins. I had no idea about horoscopes at the time, and Sanrio didn't play up that aspect of the design at all. The duo was simply a couple of kids like us, only cuter than any human could be.

Portrayals of the Little Twin Stars featured on all sorts of stationery and merchandise. In them, Kiki always floated through starry skies or against a backdrop of fluffy clouds and rainbows. His gown resembled pajamas, reinforcing in my mind his pedigree as the inhabitant of a dreamy stellar fantasyland. We were inseparable. Kiki stood on my desk, quite near where the omamori amulet had once been, watching over me while I studied. And whenever I wanted to buy something, he was there with his stock of coins.

Once a month, I'd take a few coins from Kiki, go to the bookstore in my neighborhood, and buy a copy of my favorite magazine: *My Birthday*. I'd been drawn in by the covers, which were, to preteen eyes, nothing short of spectacular. They inevitably featured an illustrated portrait of a beautiful princess of some kind, stylized not in Sanrio squishiness but in the melodramatic lines of girls' manga. But it wasn't a manga. It was a fortune-telling magazine.

You wouldn't have known it from the illustrations, which were more like fashion plates. The cover girls' enormous eyes always glimmered as though seized by some new passion. Narrow faces were framed in luxurious locks of hair parted just so to reveal gloriously bejeweled tiaras, earrings, and necklaces. The backdrops were verdant arrangements of flowers in bloom, from exotic orchids to more commonplace but equally pretty peonies and sunflowers. I don't know if I ever articulated it as such even to myself, but I can recall the emotions I felt upon seeing my first cover: *So this, this is what womanhood will be like!* It was as enticing an image of sophistication as a tween girl could possibly imagine. Every issue I bought felt like another step toward becoming one of the illustrated beauties that populated its pages.

There were articles about wholesome activities of the sort one might imagine indulging in with an idealized big sister: cooking, sewing, making potpourri. But these were mere window-dressing to the main course, which, in keeping with the magazine's name, were horoscopes.

My Birthday demystified Western-style fortune-telling with manga-style illustrations designed to put young readers at ease. Sprinkled throughout were articles on tarot cards, famous mystics, and magical incantations. Writing it out now, I realize this sounds like some sort of occult training ground for kids, but I assure you, none of its readers, or even its nonreaders, saw it that way. There was no devilry in these pages, only radiant fantasy, less dark arts than Disney princesses. And it worked. At its peak, the magazine's circulation hit 400,000 copies a month.

The magazines I read in the eighties came at the tail end of what cultural historians in Japan call our "first occult boom," which unfolded in the seventies. This was a moment when mysticism, much of it foreign, emerged from the shadows to become mainstream entertainment. The best-selling nonfiction book in Japan of 1974 was a translation of

Nostradamus's prophecies. This led to the creation of a big-budget movie adaptation produced by Toho, the same company that had unleashed *Godzilla* on global audiences. It wasn't at all uncommon to see prime-time shows featuring pseudoscience and the paranormal, from UFOs and Bigfoots to lost civilizations and haunted locations. A novelist turned politician organized an expedition to find the Loch Ness Monster, and his adventures in Scotland were widely chronicled in the mainstream media. Decades later he would become governor of Tokyo.

Mysticism was still very much in the air in the early eighties, and children such as myself embraced it with, if anything, even more gusto than the adults. After the psychic Uri Geller appeared on Japanese television, kids bent so many cafeteria spoons that schools were forced to issue "no spoon-bending" regulations. My own school's library carried numerous collections of spirit photography, and I'd sometimes hear a scream erupt from the stacks when someone discovered a particularly shocking picture. Occasionally, I will admit, the screamer was me.

My fascination with *My Birthday* slotted right into this society-wide trend. But I never thought it weird or strange. It made me smile. For instance, the magazine often contained lists of incantations called omajinai, which were akin to spells that might make little wishes come true. I remember that one in particular had instructed, "If there's a boy you like, visualize him in your mind and recite 'Zero is the letter O in love!' while dialing zero on a rotary home phone." (Fortunately, zero didn't connect you to an operator in Japan, as it did in the US.) Another was "If you want someone to become your best friend, walk in their wet footsteps."

My favorites were the illustrated guides to fairies, elves,

good witches, and dwarves from foreign folklore, with detailed instructions on how to befriend them. "Make a bed of rose petals on your desk for Rosa, the rose fairy!" Or: "Should you wish to meet Kobold, the good goblin, leave a tiny block of cheese and a spoonful of honey by a window." To me, *My Birthday* was akin to a sweet sugar cookie, with the mystical overtones like cinnamon, dusted atop for flavor. And by taking a bite, maybe, just maybe, something wonderful and fun might happen to me, like Alice finding herself in a Wonderland tea party.

Soon, however, I started to notice changes, less in the magazine than in myself. Words and phrases that didn't settle right. I quickly realized that the issue lay with the predictions and premonitions. "Today is your lucky day!," one horoscope might chirp, while "Something disappointing may happen this week" might go another. No matter how personably these tidbits were presented, they started to bother me. I was still too young to understand big concepts like "fate" or "destiny," but I gathered that these prognostications implied that my future was set.

This led to a cascade of conflicting emotions. Words like *lucky*, *unlucky*, and *happy* appeared regularly in those pages. But I'd started to notice that the writers never defined what these words meant. What did *lucky* mean, exactly? At the end of every issue were catalogs of "lucky items for little witches," by which they meant us readers. Fairy pendants and scarab brooches; Kobold-san figurines and keyholders featuring King Solomon's bearded visage; matrices of English letters hammered into metal plates, all purported to bring happiness. They changed every few months, and sold in huge numbers to readers eager to get a little luck and happiness into their lives. I never bought any of these charms, mainly because I couldn't afford them. But did the absence of these things make me any less happy? I didn't think so. The vagueness of it all stirred doubts. The magazine was still fun to page through, but more and more, I felt like it was leaving more questions unanswered than answered.

Around the time I turned twelve, *My Birthday* switched its gorgeously aspirational covers to something simpler and more cartoony, and that ended my love affair with the magazine. By this time I'd lost my fascination with fortune-telling, believing that the only one with the power to chart my future course was myself. I didn't eschew fortune-telling altogether; if a girlfriend invited me to a palm or tarot reading, I'd happily join in. That was merely a social outlet, something I did for fun. But I largely stopped actively seeking out fortunes for myself, with the exception of the ones given out at temples and shrines on New Year's.

As I grew older, though, even my thinking about these fortunes began to change. I began interpreting them in whatever way I saw fit, absorbing whatever positive elements might be there while leaving anything negative behind. I saw my interactions with fortune-telling less as relationships than flings, without any strings or commitment. A take-it-or-leave-it sort of thing.

I knew fortune-telling wasn't for me, but neither did I begrudge my friends who seemed to enjoy it. I neither sought it out nor avoided it. Yet I accepted that someone might like something I didn't, or see value in something I didn't. That was fine with me so long as we had fun together. So long as we did, I could engage with them seriously as friends, even without taking their interests personally. Looking back now, years later, I think this was the beginning of a hanshin-hangi mindset.

THE ABILITY TO BELIEVE AND DISBELIEVE SIMULTANEOUSLY
seems so natural to me, but as I grew up and began to travel
abroad, I learned this wasn't necessarily true in other cultures. I can see it even now, whenever I have the pleasure of
experiencing my homeland through the eyes of foreign
visitors.

In my experience, when young people abroad speak of
my home country, they generally frame it in terms of modernity, whether in technology or entertainment. Gadgets
and games, anime and manga, sophisticated foods, the efficient web of public transit that links our neighborhoods and
cities. They think of Tokyo, with its gleaming lights and
sights and fashion boutiques, the backdrop of so many movies and TV shows. As a Japanese person who's traveled
pretty widely, I don't think of my country as being exceptionally modern or uniquely fun, though I enjoy riding the
bullet train, and even a Tokyoite like myself has to admit
that neighborhoods like Shibuya, with its giant display
screens and wild-looking skyscrapers, can feel a little like
something out of the future. But I know that our buildings
and trains and cars and computers, all the fruits of our
modern lives, are actually built upon a thick tangle of cultural roots that aren't so clear to casual visitors: fortune-
telling and divination, "spells" and luck, threads of belief
extending back as far as history can record, and continuing
right up to the current moment. In the West, mysticism
and modernity stand in opposition, but that isn't the case
here in Japan. Not exactly.

The visit of a family member from America highlighted
how different our approaches to the concept of fortune and
luck can be. When my husband's cousin came to Japan for
the first time, we took her to Sensoji Temple in the heart of

Tokyo, a tourist hot spot for centuries. It's a fun place. A long arcade of shops and vendors of snacks and souvenirs leads through a towering gate and onto the grounds of Sensoji Temple, a grand structure with crimson walls and a gently arching rooftop. Just before you reach the temple proper, you pass through an area flanked by peculiar-looking wooden chests, each subdivided into dozens of tiny drawers, marked with its own number in Japanese calligraphic script.

My cousin asked me what they were. I told her they were for omikuji, the drawing of sacred lots. To learn your fortune, you use a hollow cylinder. It is filled with chopstick-size wooden rods that are numbered, and the lid of the cylinder has a hole in it, just big enough for a single one to escape. You lightly shake this contraption a few times to mix the contents up, then tilt it over so a rod slides out through the opening. Every cylinder contains a hundred rods, corresponding to one of a hundred drawers, each containing one of seven levels of fortune. Daikichi (great luck) is the best. Daikyo (great misfortune) is the worst.

As fate would have it, my cousin got "great luck." Her face lit up when I explained what it meant. Then I showed her mine: "great misfortune," the worst possible outcome. The smile melted, she grabbed my arm, looked into my eyes, and said, "I am so sorry." I could tell she really meant it, too.

I started laughing. "That's okay," I consoled her. "Don't worry about it. It isn't some kind of stigma! It just means there's nowhere to go but up."

I could sense her growing confusion at my reaction, so I explained that these weren't some kind of unbreakable edicts but more like tokens of advice. Even "great misfortune," despite what it sounds like, didn't really mean you were headed for a horrible fate. It just meant to be a little more careful.

"So from that standpoint," I continued, "it's actually a good thing!"

But I could tell she was even more puzzled. That's when I realized that the way Japanese and Westerners saw fortune might be different—that our entire worldviews might be different. Hanshin-hangi lets us surrender to two opposing ideas—brains telling us fortune-telling may be bogus, hearts telling us there may be something to it. But this binary opens a multiverse of possibilities, to put it in pop-cultural terms.

Omikuji is the dominant form of fortune-telling in Japan today. But in olden times, Japanese attempted to clarify their fates with forms of divination collectively called ura-nai. *Ura* means "hidden" or "behind," as in discerning the hidden intentions of the kami who affect our lives from behind the scenes. English-language dictionaries describe fortune-telling as "the act or practice of predicting the future by supernatural means." In other words, Western fortune-telling doesn't focus much on the past or present. And it succeeds or fails based on how accurate a prediction is or isn't.

Uranai, on the other hand, focuses more on the past and present than the future, for a simple reason: The future can be changed—it hasn't happened yet. This is basic cause and effect, in which every predicament is the result of something that happened to you in the past.

"In times of old in Japan, worries about the future stemmed from a fear of personal wrongdoings, or wrongdoings from previous lives," writes the author and folk historian Hiroshi Aramata. "People didn't really want to know the future; they wanted to know how to separate their current situation from their karma." To them, fortune-telling wasn't intended to foretell. It was, as Aramata puts it, "a form of verification to clarify what was happening in the here and now."

Uranai isn't intended for problems for which humans can devise solutions. It isn't supposed to preempt common sense. Nor is it a free card exempting one from making tough choices or painful decisions. That hard work of living is on you, not the kami. In fact, we have an old saying in Japanese: "Ataru mo hakke, ataranu mo hakke"—"Uranai misses as often as it hits." What might at first glance seem like a negation of uranai altogether actually means something more interesting: that uranai can both "hit" and "miss," simultaneously. You might not accept fortune-telling, but you aren't rejecting it, either, which opens you up to listening to the results of it, while giving you the ability to ignore them, too.

Think of it like that classical thought experiment from quantum physics: the paradox of Schrödinger's cat. In Schrödinger's hypothetical, a cat is placed in a sealed box with a radioactive isotope, a Geiger counter, and a device that releases poison if the Geiger counter activates. The decay of the isotope is totally random; there's no way to predict exactly when a subatomic event will occur, releasing radiation, triggering the Geiger counter, and in turn the poison. Since the box is sealed, there's no way to know at any given moment whether the cat is alive or dead. So long as it is unobserved, the only way to describe its condition is what is known as a quantum state: neither alive nor dead but both simultaneously. In essence, two opposing things are true at the same time.

Uranai is similar. The interpretations of any given prog-
nostication are equally limitless. In essence, you can pick
and choose your judgment of the outcome. Positive? Negative? A little of both? Neither? It's up to you. When I pulled
that fortune in Asakusa, innumerable causes and effects
combined in the past to bring me to that moment. Innumerable paths of possibilities stretched ahead of me. I could
easily have taken the "great misfortune" result in a very
negative way: *Oh my god, I am doomed!* But I didn't have a
panic attack, because I know the future isn't set. My future
depends on what I do and experience in the here and now.
That's how I was able to explain to my cousin that "great
misfortune" can be a good thing, too. It wasn't a white lie:
There was nowhere to go but up. That was the honest truth,
as I saw it.

In recent years, Sensoji Temple has discontinued the
practice of dispensing "great misfortunes" altogether. There
are still seven levels of fortune, but they never go as low as
"great." Of the 776 temples and shrines vending fortunes in
Tokyo, only 31 offer "great misfortune" outcomes. This
means that statistically speaking, there's only a .04 percent
chance of drawing it. The irony is that it takes a lot of luck
to land a prediction of great misfortune in Tokyo! This
makes me cherish that memory of pulling great misfortune
all the more.

Dealing with uncertainty in a flexible way, I've come to
realize, is something Japanese spirituality excels at. We're
all Schrödingers peering at the box that is life, trying to
figure out what's going on inside. Why stick to one interpretation of your fate?

"Uranai can also be seen as a kind of 'energy' to build
one's future," writes folklore professor Kazuhiko Komatsu.
"For us in the present, the future is like a blank sheet of

paper. People project the results of uranai onto this blank sheet as a guide. Then they bind themselves with whatever they projected, and take action. In this way, their image of the future becomes their reality." In my mind, this is the heart of how Japanese traditionally see divination. The question of whether your fortune comes true isn't up to the kami or Buddha; it's up to you and the actions you take to make it happen—or to avoid it. From this perspective, fortune-telling is less superstition and more like the power of positive thinking.

That is precisely why I enjoy drawing omikuji at shrines and temples. Or more accurately, I enjoy the process even more so than the result, because the act of drawing lots feels like I'm engaging in a conversation, like paying a little visit to kami territory. It's like a time-out from daily life, where I can let go and see what the fates, wherever they are, have in store. If I like what I see, I might take it. If I don't, I don't have to.

In this way I make my own fate. A hanshin-hangi mindset gives me the freedom to interpret these things however I like. That means infinite possibilities to choose from. But whether I take it or leave it, I always have respect for the forces beyond my control, as symbolized by the kami. That makes me feel as if my choices are endorsed by them. The kami have my back, so to speak. A refusal to declare belief or disbelief with regard to spiritual beings isn't selfish or disrespectful. If anything, I think it encourages affinity, even a sense of partnership. This can be useful in daily life, or on those occasions I find myself wanting to peer behind the veil of fate and fortune for whatever reason. But it can also help through difficult times. It even has the power to heal.

I KNOW THIS FROM PERSONAL EXPERIENCE. THERE WAS A time when I found myself at a personal rock-bottom, struggling through an experience so painful it was almost impossible. A kind of fortune-telling helped me process it. It wasn't that I wanted to throw myself upon the mercy of the heavens, or abdicate my responsibility to make decisions. I was enduring an unendurable situation, and I needed a tool to get me through, to give me the breathing room I needed.

My eighty-seven-year-old father was in perfect health, according to his annual checkup at the end of 2020. He lived near me, and stopped by my house on his slow but steady morning walks through the neighborhood. His memory was fading, but he remained in high spirits, and we got together regularly for family dinners.

The speed at which illness struck took all of us by total surprise. In March of 2021, he grew racked by internal pains and before long was refusing food and even water. My sister and I nursed him at his bedside, consulting with doctors by phone. Two days later his condition deteriorated to the point that we called an ambulance to the local hospital.

The problem was, they didn't want to admit him. The doctor reasoned that he'd be better off in a nursing facility; they couldn't take him just because he didn't want to eat. COVID-19 was obviously a factor as well. But none of this mattered to us. We knew our father. Two months earlier he'd been as healthy as an eighty-something man could be; now he was bedridden, groaning in pain at the slightest movement, his body shriveling. We knew something was horribly wrong. My sister all but forced the doctor to run my father's bloodwork before making a final decision.

As we waited for the results, the nurses asked us to wait

outside, a social distancing measure. I readily agreed. I needed to calm down; waves of confusion, sadness, and anger were crashing on the rocks of forty-eight hours without much sleep.

We'd been following the ambulance when we arrived, so I hadn't noticed then, but when I stepped outdoors I realized the hospital faced holy ground. A Buddhist temple and a Shinto shrine stood side by side, right across the street from the entrance. The shrine venerated a local kami. The temple honored a patron deity of healing known in Japan as Yakushi Nyorai, the Medicine Buddha.

I crossed the street and paid my respects at the shrine, bowing twice, clapping twice, bowing once. Then I did a U-turn and walked into the neighboring temple, where I bowed my head to Yakushi Nyorai. I could have used these opportunities to beg the deity to save my father. But I didn't. My father had fought hard. We all had. Now, I sensed, we were well into kami territory. The unpredictable. The unknowable.

Losing one parent had been hard enough. Losing the second was unthinkable, unimaginable. Yet it was happening before my eyes and there was nothing I could do. I didn't want to plead for his salvation. If I started down that path, I knew, the fear would seize me and never let go. It would drag me down with it. I had to be strong.

I took a deep breath. I didn't want to beg; I wanted a conversation. And I realized I had the tools to do it, tools I'd had for a very long time, forged in my experiences leading all the way back to that omamori my parents had given me as a little girl.

As I stood before the temple's altar, I devised a little uranai divination of my own. A way of intuiting the will of the heavens above. I would bow my head here and pray. If my father was accepted into the hospital, I'd see that as a "yes"—that he might live. If he wasn't accepted, I'd see it as a "no." In that case, he'd most certainly die. But I'd respect either outcome as the will of fate, no matter how devastating it might be.

These were the days of pandemic, of quarantines and restrictions of all kinds on daily life. No amount of arguing could force them to admit my father if they refused—and I knew that no other hospital would take him in, either, understaffed and overburdened as they were at this time. With my silent prayer, I left things in the hands of fate—which is to say of the kami and Buddhist deities. For whatever happened next was utterly out of my hands.

A famed swordsman by the name of Miyamoto Musashi faced a similar situation in the seventeenth century. Musashi traveled the length of Japan challenging other martial artists, and racked up sixty-one victories, all the more impressive when you remember that these contests were to the death. He survived through a combination of extraordinary skill and innovative thinking, a self-taught genius who never aligned himself with any school of martial arts.

There is a story about one of Musashi's best-known duels. Actually, *duel* isn't the right word; he was about to face down an entire school of rival swordsmen simultaneously. Even the great Musashi, undefeated in all of Japan, suspected that he would not survive this encounter. Yet honor bound him to follow through. On the way to the confrontation he passed a shrine, and instinctively went in to offer a prayer to the kami. But then he stopped:

> What am I doing? *he thought in horror.* What was I going to request? What need have I of the help of the kami?

He was appalled. Without thinking, without remembering his years of training and self-discipline, he had been on the brink of begging for supernatural assistance.

In the next breath, a wave of gratitude surged over him. The presence and magnanimity of the kami enveloped him . . . Doubt vanished; the kami had guided him to this place to teach him this.

While believing sincerely in the kami, he did not consider it the Way of the Samurai to seek their aid . . . Stepping back a pace, folding his hands, he thanked the kami for their timely help.

Musashi survived that battle and lived to see many more. But a week before his death, decades later, he gave his disciple a short text titled "The Way of the Lone One." It consists of twenty-one precepts based on his worldview and philosophy. One of the keys is the epigraph of this chapter: "Respect the kami and Buddhas, but do not depend on them."

I am not a swordsman, of course. I'm not even a martial artist. But I understand what he means. I don't cling to the kami or Buddhist deities, because I don't have to. Whenever I feel unstable, whenever it feels as though the earth is twisting beneath my feet, all I have to do is to remind myself that they are there. That is enough. They are there, somewhere, and they are watching, somehow. I may be all by myself, but I am never alone. That stirs courage.

As I prayed, the cherry blossoms were in bloom. The branches dotted with their soft flowers arched over my head and the altar before me. Now and then a petal would drift down, adding another daub to the mosaic of pale white and pink dotting the ground. Cherry blossoms are freighted with meaning in Japan: life, death, everything in between and beyond, inspiring countless poets who, like the cherries themselves, once flourished and now fertilize the soil below. But I put that out of my mind. I was facing enough loss as it is. When I looked at the delicate flowers overhead, they reminded me of Konohana-sakuya-hime, the Blossom-princess, a female kami who is the embodiment of the cherry tree. She was making herself seen here. I am struggling, I thought, but there is still beauty to be found in this world. I am frightened, but I am not alone.

I felt just a little better while walking back to the hospital. As I approached, my sister emerged from the waiting room. The results of my father's bloodwork were in. His levels were bad—critically so. It was, on the surface, terrible news. But it also meant that the hospital would have to admit him right away. A sign from the heavens? Whatever the case, he was getting another chance.

While my sister was at the receptionist desk taking care of his paperwork, I wheeled him down the corridor toward an elevator. It pained me to see my father, who had been healthy before, hunched into practically a ball, clutching the mobile IV drip stand positioned between his legs like a drowning man clutches a life preserver. Suddenly he mumbled something. I leaned over and asked him what he just said. He said thank you. I asked him why.

"If you two hadn't been around, your papa would have had to go through this all by himself."

"Well, aren't you lucky to have us for daughters?" I joked, a little desperately, in an attempt to lighten the mood. But he just gazed up at the ceiling. For a while he said nothing.

"You've been a big help," he said.

His response reminded me of long-ago conversations. My father never talked about fortunes with anyone, with one exception: me. "You keep impressing me, Hiroko," my father would say from time to time, and not in regard to any particular happening. "You seem to have a great luck in you."

Once, struck by the randomness of it, I asked him why.

"Luck is a skill," he said, which was less an answer than something else I'd heard him say many times over the years. It usually came up in the context of a certain story, or rather, a certain pattern of reminiscing. Everyone's life has its ups and downs. That's the nature of life. So it was with my father's life. He'd experienced some real lows. But inevitably, no matter how glum the situation, someone would unexpectedly emerge with advice or help. When he said this, he'd always pause for a moment right there. Sometimes he'd take a sip of green tea. Sometimes he'd look down at the half-eaten sweet on his plate. It was obvious that he was remembering. What specifically, he never said. Because then he'd look up and say the same thing. "It's just a pattern I've noticed," he'd say. "I can't explain it, but I know one thing for sure. I've been lucky. And I've always been grateful for that."

What he meant, I think, is that there's no logic to luck. If there were, it wouldn't *be* luck. It's a little like that hoary old phrase about seeing the glass as being half empty or half full. I've never liked this saying because I don't see life as an either-or. It's important to acknowledge what one doesn't have, because that's what we call "being realistic." But it's equally important to acknowledge what we *do* have, because that gives us strength when we feel beaten down or stressed out. It's like noticing a wild violet blooming at your feet while navigating a hard, rocky, slippery path. Acknowledging what we have helps stay our fears, gather our courage, and give us the fortitude to push ahead.

Easier said than done, of course. It is easy to forget what we have, because it's human nature to seek equilibrium, to adjust to the new normal, to put things out of our thoughts. But we forget the good things at our peril, for equilibrium can lead us to take things for granted. At our lowest moments, this can lead us to make things out to be much worse than they actually are. Acknowledging what you have is a skill—a skill that can help stop a slide down a negative path.

My father took energy and courage from his web of personal connections. Now I tried to take strength from the knowledge that I was helping and he knew he was being helped. It was an unfortunate situation, but there was fortune of a sort within it: the connections that had brought us to this very moment. We had made it here together.

A nurse arrived to take him to his bed. Because of the coronavirus, none of us were allowed to accompany him out of the waiting room. Our tears welled as she wheeled him through the doors to the elevator that would take him to his ward. Our parting was bittersweet. Relief at seeing him finally get the care he needed, colored by the agony of being pulled apart just when he needed us most.

The next day, miracle of miracles, we got a phone call from him. The IV had worked, it seemed. He felt much better, he said. He didn't remember the pain, or even having been bedridden. And then he did something I'd never heard him do before: He cried. He was so lonely, he said. He didn't quite understand why we couldn't be with him. I told him for the umpteenth time about COVID, knowing he wouldn't remember, then begged him to eat so he could get out and we could all be together again. He agreed to call again the next day. But it wasn't to be. He tried so hard to eat that he aspirated some of the food into a lung; this turned into pneumonia. Less than a week after he'd been admitted, and only days after our ray of hope in the form of that phone call, we found ourselves at a critical impasse again. "Come quickly," the nurse said. "He's getting weaker."

I had been practicing wearing a dress kimono that afternoon in an effort to distract myself. The call from the hospital came so suddenly that I didn't even have a chance to change. I rushed over dressed in traditional finery. This time, the hospital allowed us onto the ward to see him.

As we arrived at his bedside, my father's eyes fluttered open for a moment. "Noriko, Hiroko," he gasped. I was shocked at how wispy his voice sounded, but thankful he recognized us. Then he noticed my dress, so out of place for a hospital. "Are you going somewhere?" It was the last intelligible thing he said. We sat for a long time as his breaths grew rougher, then weaker. By nightfall he was gone.

Shortly after his passing, I decided to take a trip to a shrine I'd been wanting to visit, one known for its beautiful wisteria trellises. It had been a dark and difficult time; I wanted to see something bright, something natural, something beautiful. But there was another reason. I also wanted to say thank you to whoever it was who had blessed us with tiny, but no less important, gifts at the end. My father's last days weren't spent in pain. And equally so, we'd had the luxury of getting to say goodbye face-to-face when so many others were forced by quarantines to make their farewells over FaceTime—if they could at all.

I dressed in my finest: an antique kimono that had once been worn by my mother, and hairpins inherited from my great-aunt, the daughter of my mountain-climbing, scientist great-grandfather. I did this in the spirit of a family trip, as though we were all going out together for an afternoon stroll.

As it happened, this particular shrine offered omikuji fortunes, similar to those I'd done with my cousin in Asakusa.

On a whim, I paid for one. This time, it was Daikichi, the best fortune of all. I still have that fortune slip today. I look at it from time to time. When I do, I recall what my father said about luck, and my luck in particular.

My father's death was a crushing blow, one that could have sent me back into the depths of the darkness I'd fallen into when I lost my mother, years earlier. But I was a different person now. I had more tools in my spiritual toolbox, to put it another way.

The reason I was able to face my father's passing with as much strength as I could was precisely because of the wisdom I had gained during an even darker time, in the wake of my mother's passing. Death had been a shock, but her funeral was another, such a difficult experience that it all but robbed me of my ability to grieve for a time. The lessons I'd learned from that experience were hard indeed, but they were mine, and they'd prove helpful as my sister and I began the painful work of planning my father's funeral. One thing was sure: We wouldn't do things the way we had when my mother died.

CHAPTER 6

Curating Your Rituals: Funeral Buddhism

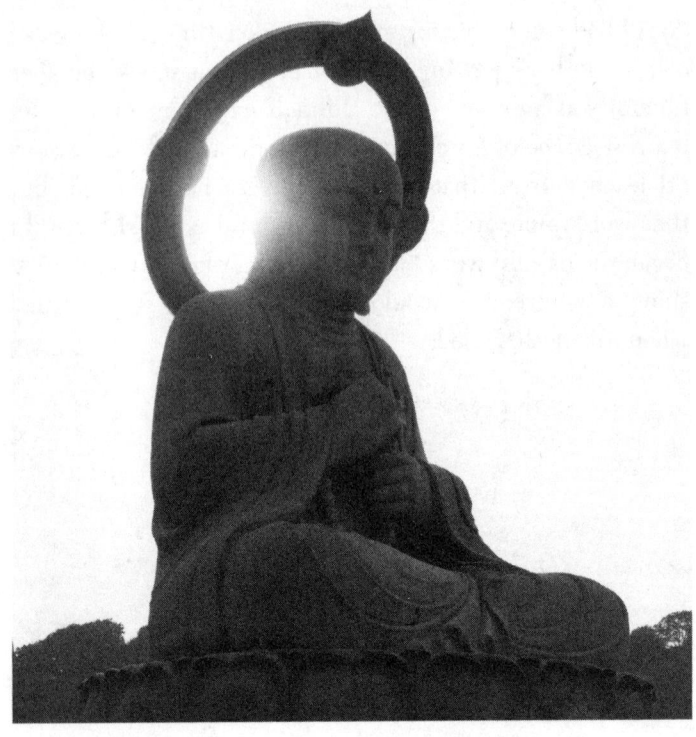

Jizo statue at Osorezan Bodaiji Temple in Aomori.

The dead don't disappear; it's just that they don't return.

—attributed to Norinaga Motoori

To die is not the end. It's a gate. You pass the gate and move
on to the next stage. As a doorman in this crematorium,
I have sent many people off, and I always say,
"have a nice trip; we'll meet again soon."

—from *Departures* (film, 2008)

When my mother died, it forced me to confront the fact that I would die someday, too. And what's more, I was told, I would have to die Buddhist. This came as much of a shock to me as my mother's passing.

"Why?" I asked my father.

"This is custom," he said. "Everyone does it that way." And so it would be.

But it didn't sit right with me. This wasn't out of any antipathy toward Buddhism. Not at all. Like many of my fellow citizens who may not consider themselves Buddhist, I still take a great deal of pleasure from Buddhist things. "Architecture, painting, sculpture, engraving, printing, gardening— in short, every art and industry that helped to make life beautiful—developed first in Japan under Buddhist teaching," wrote Lafcadio Hearn at the turn of the twentieth century, a sentiment with which I wholeheartedly agree.

I go to Buddhist temples when the opportunity presents itself, sometimes even taking in a service, letting my eyes wander over the architecture and the statuary and the altars heaped with offerings, savoring the ceremony and ritual, soothed by the rhythmic chanting of the sutras, all the while enveloped in the warm, welcoming embrace of incense. I particularly enjoy temple gardens, exquisitely composed arrangements of stone and topiary designed to evoke fundamental truths of nature. To someone born in the noise and bustle of the big city, these quiet places represent safe havens where I can collect and calm myself.

And then there is shojin ryori, literally "devotional cooking," a style derived from the strict dietary restrictions of Buddhist monks. These meals, as exquisitely composed as the gardens, consist of small dishes carefully picked to express all five tastes of sweet, sour, salty, bitter, and umami. I enjoy these meals because of their taste, but for their presentation even more. Each dish is meticulously prepared and presented so as to maximize the flavor and visual beauty of each and every fruit or vegetable, which are themselves in turn selected as complements to the seasons. Tomatoes and cucumbers refresh during summer doldrums; root vegetables like daikon radishes grow sweeter in the winter months. It is as much art as cuisine, and when I am presented with a meal like this, I feel as though I am sitting down to dine with Mother Nature herself. I almost find myself thanking every little morsel as I take a bite, for their presentations do more than delight. Eating like this reminds me of what it means to be alive.

You don't have to be a true believer to take nourishment from the things Buddhism offers, which is why so many of us do. Yet it was precisely because of these pleasant experiences that I had such a profound shock. My mother's death, or more precisely the preparations for my mother's funeral, revealed a side of Japanese spirituality I'd never known. It was as though her passing had parted a thick curtain I'd never seen, let alone thought to peer behind. What I found was what Japanese call funeral Buddhism.

I recognize that many take great comfort in Buddhist funeral traditions. But my experience with them after my mother's death forced me to confront a question I'd never before considered. What is the meaning of a ritual that brings no solace? I wrote earlier of how Japan is a rigid society with a flexible attitude toward spirituality. But for a great many modern Japanese, a Buddhist funeral represents more a social obligation than it does an expression of religious devotion. How many of us are going through the motions, culturally speaking, for reasons we barely understand?

....

I WAS THIRTY-SEVEN WHEN MY MOTHER'S LONG ILLNESS FI-nally took her from us. The loss of a parent brings almost anyone to existential reckoning. But the funeral compounded our shared grief. Most of all I remember the frustration of being coerced into doing something simply because it was considered customary, the way things were done.

My mother's passing initiated a series of Buddhist funeral rites. That was the way my father wanted it. There are 156 schools and sects of Buddhism active in Japan today, but my father didn't care much about the differences among them. He chose a Buddhist temple mainly for its convenient access. He had placed a deposit on a family plot there almost a decade earlier and had been paying an annual fee ever since. (Generally, temple gravesites are not for sale, only for rent.)

According to Japanese Buddhist tradition, a person who fails to receive a proper funeral cannot rest, and will be doomed to wander the earth for all eternity. Now, I never thought of us as a Buddhist family. I knew about the family plot, but I'd only rarely had occasions to attended Buddhist services. As sad as I was, the supposed doom of my mother's soul never occurred to me.

In the West, the image of Buddhism, especially among laypeople, is one of enlightenment and transcendence. Its influence looms large in the American zeitgeist, from gurus like D. T. Suzuki to dharma bums like Jack Kerouac and Allen Ginsberg to business mavens like Steve Jobs, forming the underpinnings of a global fascination with minimalism, meditation, and mindfulness. But you might be surprised to hear that the vast majority of Japanese actually interact with Buddhism less as a religious philosophy than as a business—specifically, the business of dying.

Funeral Buddhism is a uniquely Japanese manifestation of an ancient religious tradition. Ryosuke Okamoto, associate professor of religious studies at Hokkaido University, calls it "a textbook example of religion without worship." So why do we do it? His colleague Yoshihide Sakurai, a professor at the same university, theorizes that "the formalities of Buddhist memorial services, from the reciting of sutras to the final procession of the deceased to the crematorium, can help ease feelings of despair by giving the participants things on which to focus."

But this was not the case for me. My first encounter with the formalities proved so frustrating that it sparked a new realization. Religious traditions can support us in times of trouble, but one can let them go when they no longer serve their purpose.

As I said earlier, there's an old saying in Japan: "born Shinto, marry Christian, die Buddhist." It's customary to take one's newborn to a Shinto shrine for a blessing; a great many people choose to marry in Christian-style church wedding ceremonies; and funerals almost inevitably follow Buddhist rites. But things are not that simple in practice. Shinto, Christianity, and Buddhism all play much broader roles in society than these singular events suggest. Nevertheless, I had long seen this phrase as a symbol of the spiritual flexibility of my people. But it turns out that I wasn't quite right.

Societally speaking, there's quite a bit of freedom when it comes to the questions of where to get a child blessed and under which tradition you wish to marry. When my husband and I married in Tokyo, I chose a Christian-style ceremony held in a church-like room inside a hotel, officiated by a middle-aged American dressed like a priest. I say "church-like" because this wasn't an actual place of worship. And just before the ceremony I quietly asked the priest in English if he was ordained. "No," he replied. "I just work here." Which was fine with us. My husband just laughed. And mine was less a religious choice than an aesthetic one: I simply wanted to experience walking down the aisle to organ music while I wore a pretty white Western-style wedding gown.

But I didn't want to miss out on wearing a beautiful bridal kimono, either. So I chose to switch into a kimono for the reception, which is another fairly common thing to do in Japan. My sister, on the other hand, did the opposite: She chose to be married in Shinto style, at a shrine-like venue designed for weddings. She began in a gorgeous kimono, then switched to a bridal gown for her reception.

Weddings are a huge industry in Japan; the market is said to be around two trillion yen a year, the equivalent of almost thirteen billion US dollars. The bridal business encompasses the weddings themselves, of course, but also many associated things: catering, jewelry, hotels, flowers, and whatever else one needs to make a ceremony a success. Being a customer-facing business, it is predicated on service, meaning that participants are given wide latitude in making decisions about everything from the style of the wedding to the bouquets and such. The bride and groom are supported in whichever tradition they choose, and even the mixing and matching of traditions, as my sister and I did. The number-one goal is to make weddings happy and memorable for the participants.

Funerals are a big business in Japan, too, almost equal in size to that of the wedding industry. But there is far less leeway when it comes to choosing a tradition. In theory, people are free to choose whatever style of funeral and burial they like. In contrast to births or weddings, funerals are difficult times, often thrust upon us without warning. Most people naturally want to get through that trying moment as quickly as possible. Societal inertia means they are inevitably swept into the status quo of the Buddhist funeral. According to one survey, as recently as 2014, more than 91 percent of funerals held in Japan were Buddhist. This is changing, as we'll see, but Buddhist send-offs remain the dominant way for us to say goodbye to our loved ones.

Until the mid-nineteenth century, elaborate funerals were the exclusive purview of the aristocracy. By law, those for common folk were kept to a humble minimum and held only at night, making them quiet, almost clandestine affairs. After a simple ceremony in the home, the bereaved, close family, and neighbors formed a procession to carry the departed's remains to be buried. Throughout cities and the countryside, funeral customs, traditions, and graves took a great many forms. In some regions, the deceased were carried to their final resting places in carts; in others, they were shouldered by mourners in large boxes or barrels. (One of these barrel-shaped coffins plays a key role in the Akira Kurosawa film *Yojimbo*, letting the injured protagonist sneak off to safety.) In some places, the dead were buried in cemeteries; in others, bodies were interred in burial mounds away from habitation, while their headstones were placed closer to the village. A few places even practiced "air burials," where bodies were taken to caves and left to skeletonize, with the bones later collected and interred elsewhere.

This began to change in 1868. That's when the government instituted an ambitious Westernization plan, abolishing the social class system and, among many other reforms, removing the prohibition on daytime funerals. Now anyone who could afford to might host a lavish funeral, rivaling or even exceeding those of the former aristocracy. This made funerals more than just memorials. Now they could also be status symbols, opportunities for families to express their wealth and success.

On the one hand, the reforms represented a great democratization of funeral practices for the people of Japan. Anyone could celebrate the life and memory of their loved one in whatever way they chose. But as average funerals grew more and more elaborate, families needed more than just the help of neighbors to pull them off. Temples began offering more death-related services to their parishioners. This is the beginning of what we now know as funeral Buddhism.

THE KAIMYO WAS WHERE THINGS STARTED TO UNRAVEL for us.

Kaimyo are unique to Japanese Buddhism. They are titles bestowed upon monks and nuns as proof of their initiation into the religious order, or upon the elite to recognize their exalted status in society. But in modern times, they are widely given to the dead as new names for use in the afterlife. A kaimyo is seen as easing the transition from this life to the next, another step on the path to Buddhahood. For believers, it is something like getting your spiritual paperwork in order—a passport to the hereafter.

Since my father had chosen a Buddhist funeral, my mother needed a kaimyo to be considered properly buried. But the catch is that only monks can bestow kaimyo. Theoretically, they are given for free. But in practice, a donation is required. And the bigger the donation, the better and more prestigious the posthumous name. In premodern, feudal times, the higher your status, the longer and fancier your kaimyo became, packed with kanji characters seen as auspicious or honorific. The average Japanese kaimyo runs from six to nine characters. The longest one in history was bestowed upon the shogun Tokugawa Ieyasu, unifier of Japan, after his death in 1616. It runs nineteen characters, practically bursting with references to Buddhism, Shinto, light, peace, honor, and respect. For the lowest rungs of society, such as outcasts, a kaimyo would be short. It might contain ambiguous, negative, or even derogatory characters.

Japan is a democratic country today, but the idea of kaimyo as status symbols persists. The most prestigious and celebratory ones start at a million yen. Of course, you can always choose to "donate" less. But you'll get a shorter, less classy name in return. This has conspired to make Japanese funerals some of the most expensive in the world.

Neither I, nor any of my family, knew much about this historical background when my mother died. The need for a posthumous name was presented by my father as a sort of natural law, something that was simply *done*. But it bothered me. What's the need for changing a name? What does prestige really mean in this kind of situation? I found it hard to believe that the Buddha or anyone else would condemn anyone over a name change—particularly one that my mother didn't have any say in to begin with.

My sister, who together with her husband lived with my father and mother, took charge of the funeral arrangements. We knew that my father had started paying an annual fee to a local temple for a burial plot. But until this moment, it had been more an abstract concept than a concrete reality. When she visited the temple to discuss my mother's funeral, it was the first time either of us had ever set foot inside.

The temple was a traditional structure of dark wood and stucco, with a gently sloping, clay-tiled roof and a tidy garden in front. A small complex of buildings off to the side housed the monks and their families, alongside the administrative offices for the temple. My sister arrived in her formal best, a starched black suit, and rang the bell outside the offices.

An elderly monk answered, bald of pate and clad in black robes. Stooped by age, he stood no taller than my sister. He ushered her inside to a meeting room and had her take a seat at one end of a long table. He sat at the other. A middle-aged woman approached with cups of warm tea, which she placed in front of the monk and my sister. There was a long silence. Finally my sister spoke up. She explained that her mother had died.

"My condolences," said the old monk. "One million yen. That's the donation."

My mother had been sick for a very long time. Even with nationalized health care, her treatments had drained my long-retired father's finances. Money was tight for him, and all of us. My sister conveyed this to the monk as politely as she could.

"That doesn't cover my reading of the sutras over the body at the wake, by the way," he replied, as though he hadn't heard a thing she'd just said. Perhaps he hadn't. Tears welled in her eyes. Then the monk rose and excused himself, ending the conversation, such as it was. As he left the room, he brushed past several parishioners who bowed deeply in his wake.

As my sister sat in stunned silence, the woman who had served tea came over. "It's only a *suggested* donation," she said gently. My sister nodded, showed herself out, and returned to her car. Only after she closed the door did she let herself sob in frustration.

Hearing this story absolutely infuriated me. This didn't feel like a discussion or even a negotiation—it felt like a demand. I tried to put what she had just witnessed into some kind of perspective. To be a monk was among the most honorable and respected callings in Japanese society. Yet there was no mistaking the imperious tone with which my sister had just been addressed. And for what? For not having money to spare for a name? But when we told our father, he merely replied again that it was custom. His meek acceptance shocked me. My entrepreneurial father, a man who never raised a voice to me or my sister, but whom I'd seen absolutely erupt at people when necessary. In the end, after a lot of discussion among ourselves, and then again with the elderly monk by telephone, we agreed to pay an amount with which we all felt more comfortable.

A few days later, we received a letter from the temple. It contained my mother's kaimyo. I will never forget how crestfallen my father looked when he showed it to me. It wasn't just that it was short; the monk had also inserted a character with a double meaning. It could be read as "patience" but just as easily construed as "something to be put up with." It might not sound like much to an English speaker, but the appearances and meanings of characters are taken very seriously here. It felt like a weaselly, even cruel, thing to do to a man suffering the loss of his life partner. My father struggled for days to come up with an alternate interpretation for the character. After a long series of painful discussions together, he decided to abandon the kaimyo we had paid for. It would not be carved into the tombstone as was tradition. My mother would be buried under her living name after all.

You might ask yourself, why not simply just choose a different temple? Surely there must be other more compassionate monks out there? Unfortunately, things aren't that easy. Purchasing the rights to a grave plot essentially locks you in to using the services of the temple that hosts it. Moving a grave is a major deal, necessitating detailed explanations of why you are breaking your contract. Temples often charge significant fees for ending the relationship, and more for incidentals such as dismantling the grave. All together, they can run many thousands of dollars.

And the problem is bigger than any one monk, temple, or school of faith. In February of 2024, a man posted on Twitter of his experiences after his father's death. "Whenever I hear of someone's passing, I always think of when my father died," he wrote. "No matter how many times I asked the temple how much my father's kaimyo would cost, they'd never give me a number. Without any point of comparison, I paid fifty thousand yen. And the temple gave him a kaimyo of just one character. That resulted in my banning monks from my household for a good while." The post went viral, getting more than ninety thousand likes and being retweeted over seventeen thousand times. Thousands of people replied with sympathy and similar experiences of their own.

From what I've seen, American funeral services are usually conducted at dedicated funeral homes. In Japan, it's common to keep the dead at home until it is time to take them to the crematorium.

Normally, a wake is held within a day or two of the death. But when my sister contacted the temple again, she was told it would be almost a week before the monk could perform the first step in a Buddhist funeral, the reading of sutras over her body. A week was a long time to wait, especially given that it was mid-September and still quite hot in Tokyo. Local undertakers helped us lay my mother on a bed in the living room, then arranged pillows and blankets to make it seem as though she were sleeping. Beneath them were blocks of dry ice, exchanged daily for fresh ones as she, and all of us, waited for the temple's schedule to clear.

Finally, the day of the funeral arrived. The undertakers helped move my mother from her bed into the coffin. The vast majority of funerals in Japan are cremations, so the coffins aren't like the ornate furniture-like ones I associate with funerals abroad. Just a simple unfinished wood box and lid, with a little pair of shutters that can be opened over the face. This is how my mother was prepared to receive visitors for the wake before her funeral. Over the next hour or so, I spoke with well-wishers who arrived to pay their last respects.

I will never forget how awkward I felt when the monk arrived to read the sutras over my mother's body. It wasn't the one my sister had tangled with at the temple earlier. Dressed in black robes, with a shaved head, he kneeled before the casket with a rosary and a book of Buddhist sutras, from which he read aloud for fifteen or twenty minutes. He was pleasant enough, but this was the first time any of us had ever so much as laid eyes on this person. None of us had ever actually attended a service at his temple. We didn't have any connection beyond the plot my father had purchased; why would we? It felt like we were forced to share our home with a stranger at an excruciatingly sensitive time. And pay for the privilege, to boot.

All of it got me thinking: Why are we going through these motions, even if we don't believe? What compelled a society of people who embrace so many different spiritual ideals to orient themselves around the funeral customs of one specific religion? Much later, I'd learn something even more surprising. The ubiquity of Buddhist funerals and posthumous kaimyo names and all the rest wasn't exactly the work of Buddhists. It emerged and evolved from the arrival of what was then a new religion: Christianity.

THE MISSIONARIES ARRIVED FROM EUROPE IN 1549. ALONG with their religion they brought knowledge and medicines from abroad, and introduced new kinds of cuisine, like baked cakes and batter-fried foods. But the ships that carried them across the seas carried more troubling cargoes as well: gunpowder, and the threat of colonialism.

For a while the foreign holy men were allowed to operate fairly freely. But in 1603, the shogun Tokugawa Ieyasu grew wary of a populace who might swear loyalty to a foreign god rather than to him. He took draconian steps: banning Christianity altogether, on pain of death, then shutting Japan's borders to the outside world.

Next, he compelled the entire citizenry to register at Buddhist temples. Under the shogun's rule, Buddhism was no longer a choice but compulsory. Households were legally required to tithe money to the temples to which they were registered, and when a member died, the family was obligated to pay for a Buddhist funeral. The influx of cash expanded the influence of temples like never before, in all spheres public and private, in life and in death. Things would continue this way for two and a half centuries, until the collapse of the Tokugawa Shogunate in 1868. Today, citizens are totally free to choose their own spiritual paths, but Buddhist funerary rites remain the norm. Old habits die hard.

This might make you wonder: What about Shinto funerals? They are exceedingly rare, to the point that I have never seen one, or even heard of one being conducted among the families of my acquaintants. Surveys bear this out: just 1.4 percent of Japanese conduct funerals in the Shinto style—even less than the 1.7 percent of Christian funerals. But Buddhism's domination of the funeral sphere isn't anything new. In fact, the connection goes back to the very beginning of the religion's arrival in my country, many centuries ago.

Buddhism spread through China and Korea via the Silk Road, but it arrived in Japan over the sea, through official diplomatic exchanges. For many years after its introduction, it remained largely a tool of the emperor, for it was believed that ensuring his health and prosperity would lead to the same for the nation as a whole. Thus, the primary role of Buddhist monks in the years after Buddhism's arrival wasn't saving souls. It was carrying out rituals to ensure the protection of the imperial family from kegaré.

Kegaré is the Japanese term for spiritual pollution. The cleansing of kegaré is one of the pillars of Shinto and the purpose of its many purification rituals and ceremonies. Perhaps because kegaré is so fundamental, it is vaguely defined. Not even my Shinto Cultural Examinations textbook pins it down, attributing it to "the unpleasant feelings caused by contact with the unclean or the horrifying"—in other words, what one might call bad vibes. But long ago, kegaré was very specifically associated with the dead. Even the hint of contact with death could pollute you, and spread like a contagion to others, sickening or even killing them in turn.

At this time in history, more than a thousand years ago, the only funerals monks were allowed to officiate were those of the nobility. Aristocrats who passed away were treated to lavish Buddhist send-offs and interred in elaborately marked graves. Other castes weren't so fortunate—even those who served the aristocracy. It didn't matter if you were a faithful chamberlain, for instance, or even a monk. If you showed signs of serious illness and weren't from the aristocracy, you might be cast out, left to die far from the imperial quarters lest you pollute it or its inhabitants with the kegaré from your passing. The concept of holding funerals for commonfolk simply didn't exist, and neither did graves. Their corpses were often left where they fell, or discarded on riverbanks, or on seashores, or in forests.

A civil war in 1185 decisively shifted the power from the imperial family to the warrior class. In the wake of this shift, new schools of Buddhism emerged that better responded to the needs of samurai warriors, farmers, and townsfolk. With them came monks who didn't treat deaths as impurities; they oversaw funerals and taught their flocks that anybody, not only aristocrats but also commoners, could make it to the Pure Land simply by chanting "namu-amida-butsu"—"I trust in the merciful Buddha." In an era of warring states, civil war, and endless disasters natural and man-made, the idea that anyone could make it into heaven understandably resonated throughout the populace. In many ways it was a time of death, and the Buddhists' embrace of it, in the sense of helping comfort the bereaved, made them pillars of society. The rituals and ceremonies they developed for guiding ordinary folks into the hereafter represent the foundation of modern-day funeral Buddhism in Japan.

Shinto served many needs in communities of the era, but its abhorrence of death meant that it lacked the tools for funerals. Its rituals focused on purifications—and those were cold comfort to those grieving over the loss of their loved ones.

The pioneering folklorist Kunio Yanagita was the son of a Shinto priest and wrote of his experience with Shinto funerals. "The problem with Shinto," he wrote in an essay published in the 1940s, "is that it lacks chants designed for funerals specifically." Yanagita confronted this head-on when his father passed away in 1929. For the funeral, the local priest performed what is known as a Grand Purification. This rite is a pillar of Shinto. Its chants invoke "all the eight million kami in the heavens above and on the Earth below," beseeching them to "drive away," "blow away," and "swallow" any and all forms of kegaré, then "seal them away in an unknown place." It isn't designed for sending off the dead but rather to drive impurities from sacred spaces.

"Repurposing this chant for last rites creates a sense of unease among the gathered," wrote Yanagita. "During my father's funeral, I was too emotionally drained by my grief to pay much notice. But when the priest conducted the ceremony again, on the anniversary of his passing a year later, it was pure agony. For I wanted his soul to linger even just a little longer."

Given that Shinto traditionally treats the dead as sources of kegaré, it's easy to sympathize with Yanagita's mixed feelings about Shinto funerals. Listening to a chant designed to drive spirits out when one is in the midst of deep grief, he wrote "was almost too much to bear."

Stung by this experience, Yanagita asked local priests if they might compose Shinto chants more suitable for the deceased and their loved ones. But he found no takers, for "back then, in the countryside of Chiba where I lived, even many Shinto priests were given Buddhist funerals when they died." Eventually, he experimented with creating several of his own, which he used in private remembrances. Unfortunately, they're lost to time, but as he wrote of these efforts, "I like to think they brought my father some pleasure." I like to think so, too.

As Japan's economy boomed in the postwar era, funerals grew more and more extravagant. In one notorious instance, a multimillionaire paper magnate by the name of Ryoei Saito paid record-setting prices for Vincent van Gogh's *Portrait of Doctor Gachet* and Renoir's *Dance at Le Moulin de la Galette* at auction in 1990, then sparked international fury by declaring his intention to have them cremated with him when he died. (After Saito's passing in 1996, his family wisely declined to follow through on his wishes.)

Even after Japan's economy crashed in 1990, the lure of flashy funerals continued. In a survey from 2007—almost two decades of recession later—the average cost of a funeral was reported to be well over two million yen, something like seventeen thousand US dollars at contemporary exchange rates, the highest in the world. By comparison, the cost of launching one's remains into orbit aboard a rocket that same year was "only" one million yen. It cost literally twice as much to be buried Buddhist as it did to go into space.

But today, Japan is no longer as wealthy as it once was. People live longer, and a declining birth rate means there are fewer people in general. Many households consist of just one or two members. And modern gig-economy urban life is not conducive to fostering community ties. It is not at all uncommon for people to experience what is called kodoku-shi, a solitary death.

This has led critics to publicly question why funerals are so expensive in Japan. And people seem to be listening: In 2010, a book whose title translates into *Funerals Are Not Necessary* hit the bestseller list. Technology is also disrupting tradition in unexpected ways, such as when an enterprising funeral firm began "delivering" monks via Amazon for a fixed price in 2015. Increasing numbers of Japanese are reducing the role of religious leaders in their funerals, or even excluding them altogether.

The pandemic accelerated the trend. For several years, restrictions on gatherings precluded large-scale funerals of any kind. But even putting aside infection concerns, more and more people are choosing to make their own funeral traditions—a trend local observers have called "the individualization of death." When the husband of a celebrity chef died in 2019, she made waves by telling mourners to wear jeans instead of a traditional funeral dress and filling her husband's casket with his favorite foods. And she made a point of not involving monks. Rather than sutras, she played Frank Sinatra.

Thanks to Japan's long history with Shinto and Buddhism, locals have been mixing and matching religious beliefs for a very long time. Some of these practices have codified into a sort of conventional wisdom that's tempting to call common sense. But after my mother's and father's deaths, I realized that there's no need to bind oneself to tradition. Beliefs and practices are options to be considered and chosen. It is perfectly fine to have a Buddhist funeral if you take solace in those traditions. But at the same time, it is also perfectly acceptable to have a nondenominational or even entirely secular one. We have the power to define our choices.

....

THE ONE-YEAR ANNIVERSARY OF MY MOTHER'S PASSING was rapidly approaching. Traditionally, families hold a small graveside service to commemorate the date of their loved one's passing every year. Some schools of Buddhism suggest holding them annually for thirty-three years, while others promote as many as fifty. Each service involves another obligatory donation for a monk to light sticks of incense and read sutras over the grave.

In the end, my father negotiated with the temple for a pair of new kaimyo: one for my mother, and another for himself, for when the time came. Having no more money to spare for a donation, he offered his services instead, helping sweep the grounds and writing occasional articles for the temple's newsletter.

"Is this really necessary?" I asked him. He said that it was. It drove home to me just how important the idea was to his generation. And if it brought him peace, I was all for it.

But we decided not to involve the temple directly in our grieving anymore. When the anniversary came, we didn't enlist the monks for a ceremony. We went to the grave as a family, by ourselves. My father read the Heart Sutra over her grave himself. Then we returned home, had sushi delivered, and ate, drank, and shared memories of my mother. This turned into a new annual family tradition of its own. We would go to the temple several times a year to place flowers on her grave. First we would visit the temple's prayer hall, to thank the Buddha and the temple for watching over my mother, and then we would clean her headstone, as is customary. At these times my American husband, who of course joined us on these sojourns, would bow his head and pray right alongside us. Neither he nor I identified as Buddhist. But it didn't matter. We did not see these visits as religious observances. Our prayers to the Buddha were a matter of custom and respect, more than personal faith. The visits weren't religious with a capital R. They were about seeing mother, and supporting one another. Remembering someone in the way you think they would want to be remembered brings you closer to them. It's like weaving something substantial out of an ethereal memory.

When my father passed away at the age of eighty-eight in April 2021, my sister and I again chose to grieve in our own way. We would conduct the wake ourselves, just the closest five family members, with no monk at all.

We retained the services of a local undertaker to assist us with the logistics of bringing the body back home to prepare it for the cremation a few days later. On his twin bed we laid him out, just as we had my mother on hers more than a decade before. Working together with the advice of the undertaker, my sister and I got him out of his hospital robes and into a dress shirt and pants. We arranged him on the bed and pulled the comforter up to his chin. He would stay here, cooled by dry ice, until the cremation a few days later.

On the day of the service, staff arrived to help us transfer my father from his bed into his casket. They provided trays of flowers for us to arrange inside, and encouraged us to place mementos inside for him to "take with him." First we put in the wooden walking stick that he'd relied on for so many years, so that he would have it if he needed it, wherever he was going. We laid his old tuxedo atop him, and his favorite dress shoes by his feet. Atop his legs we laid my mother's dress, the same one she'd worn on a trip to Europe together with him in 1989. He'd taken her there to cheer her up after my sister and I had left home to study in the States. A photo of the two of them taken there was one of his most cherished possessions to the end, and now, we thought, he could re-create it with her, when they reunited on the other side. My husband slipped in a plastic flask filled with my father's favorite single-malt Scotch. My sister slid a package of tissues into his pocket, for he was always asking her for a pack whenever he left the house. And at the last, I placed a family photo we'd taken on New Year's Day. My father was still healthy then, and all of us smiled in front of a traditional meal, celebrating the start of the new year. I knew he'd want it, wherever he was going, to show off with pride to anyone he might meet.

To us, this was more than a ritual or even a formality. We approached it with all the seriousness we would have had he been going on a journey in life. It would be the very last time we could help him go somewhere.

When we finished, the head undertaker turned to us and asked what sect my father had been. All of us paused. Then, one of us responded "Pure Land Buddhism," because that was the sect of the temple where he'd paid for the family grave. But then again, he'd only become a member by virtue of purchasing a grave there. Did that make him a believer? He'd chosen a Pure Land temple. But none of us had ever really spoken about Buddhism, let alone this particular sect.

The undertaker told us to put our palms together and re-cite the phrase "namu-amida-butsu" together. It is one of the most famous chants in Japan, a plea to the Buddha for safety and salvation, something like the "Hail Mary" in Christian practice. We quietly intoned it several times together. If this was intended to stir any religious epiphany within me, it wasn't working. The unaccustomed chant sounded like a foreign language. When we were done with this impromptu ceremony, the undertaker spoke up again.

"He's already in Pure Land—straight to heaven, just like that."

The words were meant kindly, and I took them as such. But they also struck me. Logically, I knew the man was merely explaining what Pure Land adherents believe happens to a soul after its owner dies. To them "namu-amida-butsu" is more than a prayer; it is almost like a magical spell, with the power to transport a loved one to the hereafter. The chant brought its believers great peace, and I would never begrudge anyone that. But what solace does it give nonbelievers such as myself? The philosophy of a religious tradition in which I didn't participate certainly didn't assuage my grief.

In Japan, there are many variations of the form the afterlife takes. As far back as elementary school, I recall a teacher saying that she thought our souls went back to wherever they came from before we were born. The Pure Land sect holds that the world of the departed lies far to the west; in Okinawan lore, it is far to the east in a realm known as Nirai-kanai. Monks of the Tendai sect of Buddhism once set sail into the sea, hoping they might reach their own school's promised land in the south. And Shinto places its underworld underground, far beneath our feet, in the form of Yomi-no-kuni. The point is nobody knows. The only thing linking them is the fact that once people die, they are no longer part of our world. They depart the realm of the living. They are forever beyond our reach.

I was standing in front of a coffin, my father's cold body lying inside. There was no way any religious philosophy could be more profound than that. Or so I told myself, but in truth I was struggling to hold myself together in the face of another, even more brutal reality. In just a few hours, we would be at the crematorium.

It was the middle of spring and the cherries were at full blossom, but a cold rain fell as we followed the hearse by car. My brother-in-law drove; my husband sat in the front seat; and my sister and I sat in the back, with her eleven-year-old daughter between. The ceremonial room in the crematorium was large, about half the size of a high school gymnasium, perhaps, with numerous furnaces capable of holding several funerals simultaneously. But this was in the midst of Japan's first wave of COVID-19 cases, and we had the cavernous room almost entirely to ourselves. It was just us; the undertaker; his associate, who had wheeled my father's casket inside; and a crematorium employee dressed in white trousers and work jacket, topped by a hat reminiscent of a chauffeur's. This man opened a pair of shutters at the head of the coffin so we could see father's face one last time. Then it was time to let him go.

The worker pushed the casket to the edge of a conveyor belt of rollers, then pressed a button to open the furnace. We stepped back as the coffin rolled inside the chamber. Everything was conducted with an efficiency borne of respect for the bereaved, and countless repetitions. The heavy steel doors slid shut. My husband gripped my hand tightly and I gripped back, my legs jelly, my eyes blurred with tears, afraid I might collapse. There was a loud *woosh*. Through a tiny porthole in the door, I could see the flames lick up. Instinctively, I clasped a hand over my mouth, because I knew, knew, that if I didn't, I would scream.

"There is no sadness greater than the inevitable journey of death," wrote the philosopher Motoori Norinaga in the eighteenth century. "Confucianism and Buddhism use various pretexts to assuage our sorrows. But there is no way to equivocate with death. Any story that attempts to temper our despair cannot be the true path." I thought of these words as we sat in the waiting room. After lighting the furnace, the staff had ushered us here, for it would take a half hour for my father to be reduced to ash. We sat in silence, drained from the events of the previous few days.

I had spent the night before at my father's house, in our old living room, on a sofa next to the bed he'd moved there when my mother first grew too ill to climb the stairs. When we brought his body home, the bed became his bier. Following tradition, we laid him not as he slept in life, but in the opposite direction, his head facing north. Later I would learn that this common practice, known as kita-makura, literally "north-pillow," was another adoption from Buddhism, which holds that this is the way the Buddha was laid out when he passed. But at the time, like most Japanese, we had no idea of these origins. We were merely following custom.

The funeral company had placed a small altar, about a foot high and two wide, next to it. Atop this sat a Buddhist prayer bell and a censer for lighting sticks of incense, which we did every morning. I'd visited every day leading up to the funeral, to help my sister with arrangements and just spend time together. But as the funeral date approached, I found myself wanting to spend one last night under the same roof with him.

My sister gave me a thick blanket to make sure that I would be warm enough, as we couldn't run the heat with his body here. I tossed and turned for many hours before finally drifting off to sleep. And as I slept I had a dream.

I was lying on the sofa, just as in real life. But in my

dream it was daytime, bright and sunny. I could hear birds chirping outside. Through the sliding-glass doors leading out of the room, I could see the garden he had tended in better times, long since gone to seed, now suddenly lush and green and in full bloom. I stood up and walked over to his bed. He was lying there, just as he was when I'd gone to sleep. I peered at his face for the last time.

Suddenly his eyes opened. With dream logic he was instantly sitting upright, facing me, haloed in warm sunlight, no longer wan and sickly but idealized and untouched by illness or the ravages of time, the father of my memories, of my heart, as I remembered him and always would. "Time for your papa to go," he said with a smile.

I awoke with a start. It was cold and dark still, and I could hear the gentle patter of rain outside. A faint scent of incense hung in the air. I snapped on the light, then raised myself on an elbow to look at my father. He was motionless, of course. On the floor by his head stood a tall vase with a spray of lilies, a popular Oriental hybrid called the Casa Blanca. I had seen them at the grocery store and brought them here the day after my father died, to brighten up the room a little. Only one had bloomed; the buds of the other three stalks remained tightly shut. I knew well enough from my own experience gardening that lilies were a fickle flower. *Wouldn't it be sad*, I thought, *if they didn't bloom at all?*

The urn containing my father's ashes was still warm as my brother-in-law drove us home. In the back seat of the car, my sister and I took turns holding it, feeling the residual heat ebb away in the cold spring air. I don't remember much about the drive, or even much of that day, save one thing. When we got home and returned to the now-empty bed where my father had lain, I found that another of the lilies had unexpectedly bloomed while we were out. It was fresh and beautiful, white petals folding back to reveal the distinctive maroon-colored pistils within. It was impossible not to see this as some kind of sign.

I don't know where my father went, but wherever it is, I don't think Buddhist kaimyo or funerals of any spiritual stripe paved the way. He is somewhere, I believe, but wherever it is, it is not here. That loss is what I am grieving now, and will continue to do until I inevitably join him again, when my time comes. That is the only truth that matters.

....

MY FATHER TOLD ME THAT I WOULD BE BURIED BUDDHIST, because that was the way things were. He didn't mean this in a domineering way. He saw it following the tradition as a form of social grace. But traditions are made by people. What worked for him did not for me. So I began constructing new traditions of my own.

People have been wrestling with the aftermath of death for as long as there have been people, of course. Every society and culture has its own approaches to saying goodbye, to mourning, to healing. But I still think my country has a unique set of attitudes surrounding death, not so much in their particulars but in the way they integrate opposing notions of ancient and modern. We grow up regularly visiting graveyards, as I've mentioned I did with those family gatherings of summers past. In summer festivals we dance alongside the dead, and with altars we welcome them into our homes. Death here isn't a gulf so much as a gate. Our rituals are the attempts to help us meet the departed, at a halfway point.

The question isn't about which rituals are right; it's a question of which rituals are right for you. My mother's funeral felt as though I had tumbled into some morass, trapped in mud so thick that every step felt as though I were being drawn deeper in. No matter how I twisted and thrashed to free myself, the struggle only served to make escape feel even more impossible. No matter how loudly I screamed for help, the sounds were swallowed by the inky depths. Such was the pull of the rituals to which I felt bound. All I wanted to do was mourn my mother. But ritual in this case proved a hindrance rather than a help.

Unable to escape, I decided to take the opposite approach and dive deeper. This was the beginning of my journey into the heart of Japanese spirituality. And in those depths I discovered something. A funeral is not a form of healing. It's a farewell, which is a different thing altogether. Funerals are important, but they end, and the pain continues. And continues. How to live with that? My hunger to reunite with my parents cut like a knife. But I was starting to realize that same hunger could also be a beacon toward healing.

Nothing can erase the pain of loss. It delineates a before and after, where things are never the same again. That grief I will take to my own grave. But I discovered a way to soothe it, to help transform from open wound to scar, from something that causes pain to something that testifies to our love, something that helps us live. It is neither explicitly religious nor purely secular, but it plays a major role in Japanese life, in how we deal with loss, and how we heal from it. It's called kuyo.

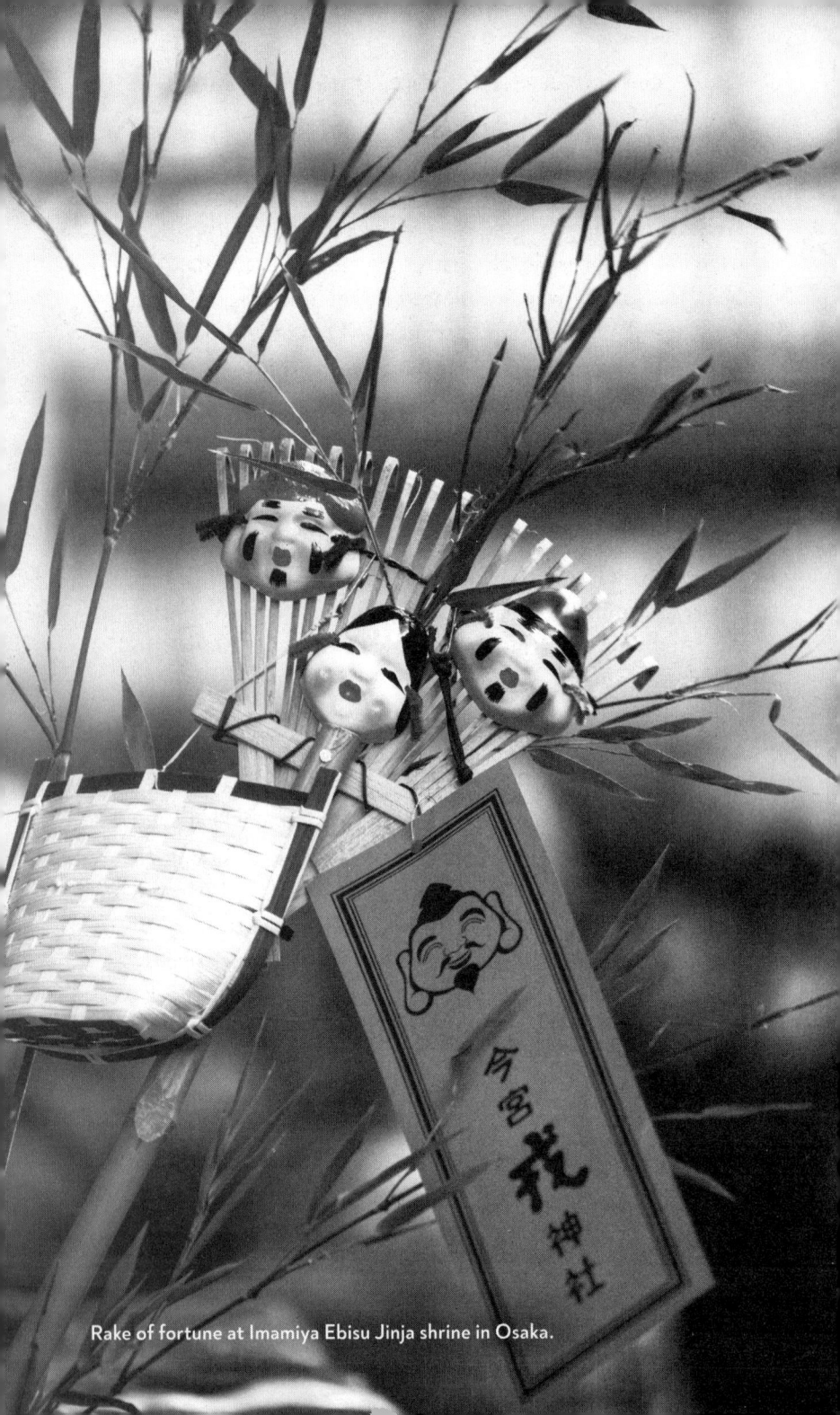

今宮 花 神社

Rake of fortune at Imamiya Ebisu Jinja shrine in Osaka.

Part Three

REBIRTH: EVERYDAY SPIRITUALITY

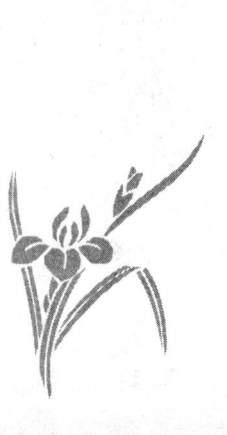

CHAPTER 7

Love Will Travel: Kuyo

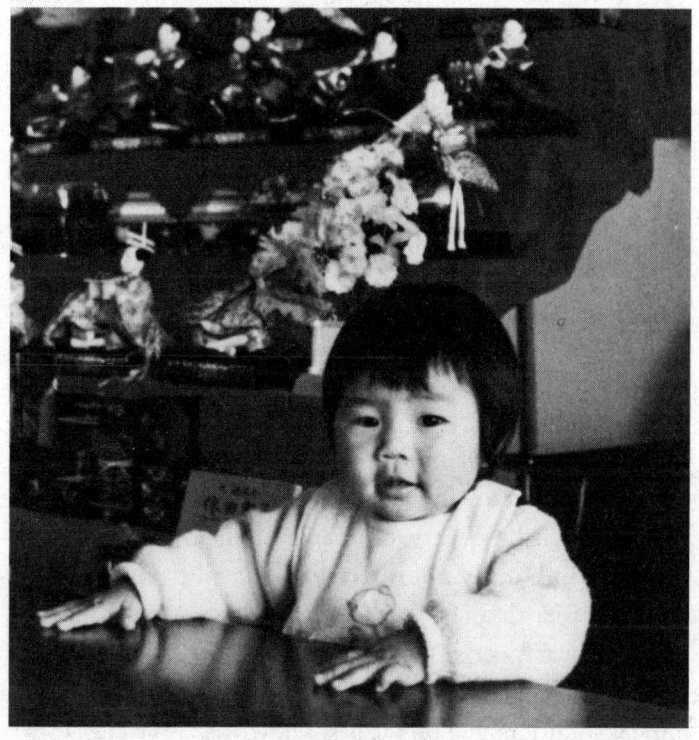

Me, at eleven months old.

A little Japanese girl does not break her doll. No, she takes great care of it, and keeps it even after she becomes a woman and is married. When she becomes a mother, and has a daughter, she gives the doll to that little daughter.

—Lafcadio Hearn

Awashima Shrine serves a tiny fishing village at the tip of a peninsula jutting into Osaka Bay. The back of the shrine faces the ocean; when you pray here, you are praying to the sea. The structure's scarlet-painted wooden rafters and pillars contrast beautifully against the weather-beaten green patina of the copper roof and the white stucco walls. On one side stretches a hillside of evergreen foliage, and on the other, the waters of the bay, slate gray under an early spring sky. But to me, the shrine's most arresting feature isn't its architecture or its location. It is the tiny faces of countless dolls, piled dozens high inside the sanctum, many more lined up in neat rows under the portico.

These are hina. They are exquisite figurines clad in kimonos, with porcelain skin and carefully coiffed hair. I've never seen so many in one place. Later a priest will tell me there are easily twenty thousand of them, some carried here by hand, many more arriving by mail from across the country. But they are not here for decoration. They are waiting for a funeral: their own.

Hina dolls play the central role in the Hina-matsuri, an annual tradition held on what is known as Girl's Day, every March 3. Whenever a daughter is born, it is customary for parents to buy a set of hina to celebrate. Basic sets include just an emperor and empress, he with a tall headdress and sword, she with a tiara and folding fan. More expensive sets add a few rows of attendants. The most elaborate feature is seven tiers of royal ministers, servants, and musicians, augmented by palanquins and oxcarts, arrayed atop bright red felt cascading over stair-stepped displays. The scene is supposed to evoke a traditional wedding procession. Capturing this festive and auspicious moment in miniature represents wishes for a child's health and future happiness.

My parents must have been quite proud of my birth, for they purchased a seven-tiered set to commemorate it. I remember the fanfare of their assembling it every spring. It was stored in a series of large boxes, each containing many smaller ones within. After carrying these down from the attic, my parents would first assemble the stand and drape it in its soft felt cover. Next, they would carefully extract the dolls from their cradles of tissue paper, and painstakingly arrange them on the tiers alongside tiny treasures: pastel slabs of faux sweets on Lilliputian lacquerware; tiny tea sets that my little sister and I would sometimes dig out during the year for our own doll tea parties; sets of dowry chests; luxurious royal litters and carts to convey the betrothed; miniature tachibana orange and peach trees, as accents. Then, after a few weeks, the process would be reversed, and the tiny retinue would return to their boxes to wait for another Girl's Day to roll around.

Until one year it didn't. Sometime after my sister and I reached our early teens, my parents stopped assembling the set. This moment came and passed without comment; to be honest, I don't think my sister and I even noticed. For years after, decades really, the dolls sat in their boxes in the attic, all but forgotten.

This might sound a little sad, but it's really a very common story. Long ago, hina dolls were treated as family heirlooms, to be passed down through the generations, but today they're more of a commodity. The role of the hina ends when a little girl grows up, and we had grown up. At some point, many families reconnect with their hina sets during a decluttering, or moving of houses, or downsizing. The boxes are rediscovered, and maybe they're even opened and cooed over again. But then what?

It's a hard decision. Few families are willing to throw hina sets away with the trash. They were expensive. They were, and still are, beautiful. And they're freighted with meaning and memory and nostalgia. Little guardian angels who shielded one's children from harm or misfortune—it simply wouldn't do to toss them with the usual food scraps and waste. So we feel a deep desire, even a need, to treat them with respect out of gratitude for their long years of companionship.

This is the service that Awashima Jinja provides. The ritual is called kuyo, and more specifically here, "ningyo kuyo"—a "doll memorial." They aren't the only ones doing it in Japan, but they are the biggest and best known.

Kuyo is written with characters meaning "offer" and "nourish." And this is just what it is: an offering that sustains a relationship beyond the grave. There are no hard-and-fast rules as to what constitutes a kuyo. Like love, you just know it when you see it or feel it. When people hold funerals, it is a form of kuyo. When they light incense sticks in memory of a departed family member, it is a form of kuyo. When the protagonists of Haruki Murakami's novel *Norwegian Wood* commemorate the life of a departed friend by playing guitar, drinking wine, and lighting matches instead of incense, that is a form of kuyo, too. A kuyo is nothing more or less than a ritualized act of love. The details are entirely up to each and every one of us. In making a ritual out of love, we reaffirm and even amplify it.

The concept is so fundamental, such a part of the fabric of daily life, that generations of native and non-native speakers have struggled to translate it into English. Most often it is "memorial service," which feels too limiting, too stiff, for acts that can just as easily be as casual as they can be formal. I've seen *Kuyo* rendered as "ancestor worship," or in older, less enlightened texts, "the cult of the ancestor." This phrasing frames it as superstitious, primitive, uncivilized. But to me, it is exactly the opposite: down-to-earth, entirely compatible with modern life, even universal; a desire to express our love and affection, our respect, to those upon whom we depend, even after they're gone. Perhaps especially after they're gone, when the realization of what we've lost hits us again and again.

I've also heard it described as Confucian, that Chinese import that stresses deference: of child to parent, woman to man, and citizen to ruler. Maybe it was, centuries ago. But Confucianism is far too reductive to explain the varied ways in which kuyo is performed today: not only for family, but for friends, for pets—even for things.

At a Buddhist temple on the bank of Shinobazu Pond in Tokyo's Ueno Park, there are kuyo-to, stone memorials, to eyeglasses and sewing needles. In the neighborhood of Tsukiji, where the city's wholesale fish market used to be, is a little Shinto shrine with memorials for eggs, fish, and seaweed. This isn't "worship" but recognition, acknowledgment, appreciation. In our mass-produced consumer society, where virtually anything we need is available at the click of a mouse button, it is easy to forget how much we depend on the things we use to make it through our days. Where would we be without glasses helping us see, needles helping keep us clothed, and the plant and animal worlds keeping us nourished? Memorials like this are quiet reminders from the past, telling us to stop for a moment, and remember where we came from.

Kuyo even inflects the way we speak. In Japan it is unthinkable to begin a meal without saying "itadakimasu"—a word that means "humbly receiving with gratitude," but note the lack of a specific subject. We are receiving the food from whoever prepared it, but also from whoever cultivated it, and finally whatever sacrificed itself so that we could have it. "Itadakimasu" reminds us of the invisible web of relationships upon which we rely to live.

"No man is an island," the seventeenth-century English poem goes. "Any man's death diminishes me, for I am involved in mankind." It's a beautiful sentiment, and Japanese spirituality takes it a step further. None of us is an island, and neither is humanity as a whole. In an animist's world, where everyone and everything has a spirit, our "involvement" goes far beyond ourselves. This is how kuyo evolved over the centuries, from memorializing the aristocratic elite—its earliest form—into commemorating one's relatives, and then into celebrating the things that support us throughout our lives, like animals and plants, even tools, even dolls. Kuyo isn't superstitious, uncivilized, or cultish. It's a celebration of everything that makes life worth living.

If you looked at that mountain of hina dolls at Awashima Jinja with the right eyes, you might see tens of thousands of invisible threads, each tallying a birth, each linked to a little girl who had long since grown up into a woman. These faithful little hina had been there at the start, watching over those lives. The presence of so many dolls here today spoke to the profound reality of those connections forged decades ago.

A small crowd, mostly women, had gathered outside the

shrine by the time the service began. On the portico sat three small boats, each perhaps a third the size of a canoe, assembled from fresh, unfinished wood. Plain wood is widely used in Shinto structures and rituals, a representation of nature in its untouched form. Each boat was decorated with pink peach tree branches, in full bloom at the season, and yellow canola flowers.

For several minutes, the priest recited a Shinto prayer. Then a boy and a girl dressed in traditional Shinto robes began picking dolls out of the pile. They took turns holding each up to the crowd and describing it—for instance, "Odairi-sama desu," "This is an emperor," the act of recognizing it by name one final time, another reminder of the role it, and all of these dolls, once played in someone's life. Then they would carefully nestle it inside one of the boats. Other children had been enlisted to toss paper confetti as this was going on, showering the proceedings with tiny flashes of color.

Each boat held about 150 dolls. These would stand in for the rest. A pair of wooden bars extended beneath each hull, allowing the vessels to be shouldered and carried, like the portable mikoshi shrines used in neighborhood festivals. The priest encouraged the women in the audience to help carry the boats to the water, where the hina would be launched off on their final departure. There were too many of us to carry the boats at once, so we took turns. As mine came around, the procession was already nearing the beach. Suddenly a wind blew in from the ocean. The confetti that had settled atop the dolls leapt into the sky, then swirled down like snow all around us. I felt a piece alight in my hair, which I took as the pat of a tiny hand, thanking me for my efforts.

We lined up the boats on the beach, a dry spot just beyond where the waters lapped into the sand before retreating back into the bay. The priest recited another Shinto prayer, asking the kami to receive these gentle hina with open hands. Local fisherfolk released each boat into the waves. As the last floated away from shore, carried by currents to the beyond, the public ceremony drew to a close. The remaining dolls would be cremated on pyres over the days to come.

There were many teary eyes in the crowd as we dispersed. I understood. My dolls weren't among the ones given a send-off on this day; those still remained ensconced in the attic of my childhood home. I'd come to the ceremony out of pure curiosity. But participating in it rekindled old memories that had been tucked away in the rafters of my mind. Something precious, something I'd taken for granted, even forgotten: How happy my parents must have been when I was born. I'd been living on my own for many years by this point, but even after becoming independent, I depended on them in many other ways, large and small. They were gone now, but I would have never gotten where I was without them. In that way they were still with me.

I always associated Shinto with celebratory rituals, such as births, and Buddhism for more somber ones, such as funerals. And it's true that Buddhist temples conduct the lion's share of kuyo rituals, for both people and objects. But here in Awashima was a Shinto shrine doing the exact same kind of thing. On the one hand it felt akin to seeing a menorah in a church. But this was more than an exception that proved the rule—it felt like the rule itself. That kuyo, the way in which we interact with the dead, transcends religion. It isn't secular, but neither is it specifically religious. It's fundamental to Japanese culture, but nobody sees it as an affiliation or identity. It's just something one does, when the opportunity presents itself. Kuyo is a ritualized form of expressing gratitude, but it's something more: a wish that your love will travel, transcending borders and realms of existence to reach whoever or whatever it is you want to touch with your feelings of gratitude. This is what makes kuyo so difficult to explain to those not raised with it.

I suspect this is why Marie Kondo's advice to thank one's belongings before disposing of them seems to evoke such shock, even distaste, among Westerners. Now, I don't thank my old clothes before parting with them, but I get where Kondo is coming from. Would *The Guardian* have described her as "woo-woo nonsense," or *The New Yorker* have called her a "freelance exorcist," if they understood kuyo?

....

JAPAN REGULARLY APPEARS ON LISTS OF THE LEAST RELI-gious countries. According to statistics compiled by the Japanese government's Agency for Cultural Affairs, around 180,000 groups are legally registered as religious organizations. Together, these groups claim about 180 million followers—a startling figure, given that Japan's population is only 125 million. In an accompanying report, the agency theorized that the official numbers of followers were inflated by what it called citizens' "weak sense of religious belonging." In English, this sounds like some sort of deficiency, a lack of spiritual conviction. But in reality, it depicts the polar opposite: that large numbers of Japanese felt comfortable claiming a relationship with multiple faiths simultaneously. It means few see any one religion as their identity.

My graduate work in International Peace and Conflict Resolution took me to religious places around the world. Those experiences gave me the sense that Westerners tend to be born one thing, religiously speaking, and then over the course of their lives either stay that way, convert, or quit outright. The acts of committing to another faith, or abandoning it altogether, represent major life moments. Even simply being un-religious can take on heavy connotations, such as how atheism can represent a powerful form of identity among those who claim it.

The Japanese experience is almost the opposite. We have no shortage of religious choices either, but relatively few of us choose to specifically identify with any one. Honestly, the idea doesn't really even occur to us—it certainly never did to me, or any of my family or friends. We never discussed religion among ourselves. Many of our spiritual traditions, like kuyo, are so quotidian that we barely even notice them in the act. This is why in survey after survey, some 70 to 80 percent of Japanese citizens profess to having no religious beliefs at all.

Part of the problem is the question of what constitutes religious beliefs, or even religion. It might surprise you to learn that the translation of the term *religion* (shukyo) is of quite recent origin, dating only to the late nineteenth century. After America's gunboat diplomacy opened Japan's ports to the world, in 1858, many locals saw how our "hodgepodge" spirituality, as one Japanese religious leader termed it, stood in contrast to the organized, evangelical religions of the West, where one's faith hinged on a contract with an almighty God.

This absolutism perplexed the polytheistic Japanese. Scholars of the time grappled with "religion" alongside other imported concepts, such as "liberty," "individual," "constitution," and "bank." The idea of shukyo effectively pitted Japan's agrarian spiritual traditions, and by extension Japan itself, against the ascendant industrial West. In books and lectures, critics argued fiercely about whether Shinto and Buddhism represented shukyo or something altogether different.

The discussion doesn't really happen anymore. While academics debated among themselves, average Japanese citizens simply went about their hodgepodge spiritual lives as usual. In essence, they answered the question themselves—with a collective shrug. Unencumbered by the shackles of religious identity, and surrounded by spiritual traditions of all kinds, they felt no need to play favorites, establish hierarchies, or even declare loyalty to any given one.

The reason so many Japanese answer "no" when asked if they have a shukyo—which is to say, if they're religious—is because, in our minds, the word *shukyo* itself is so intimately connected with the foreign religions that sparked the need to coin the word in the first place a century and a half ago. It is evangelism, more than belief or doctrine, that gives Japanese pause. In a 2024 survey, 83 percent of Japanese agreed with the statement that "it is unacceptable for a person to try to persuade others to join his or her religion." Muddying the waters is that the related term *shin shukyo*, or "new religions," also encompasses what would be known as cults abroad. This complicated history conspires to make discussions of religion a minefield in Japan: something preferably avoided, and requiring delicate navigation.

In my experience, most Japanese people have no issue discussing spirituality in broad terms. But the moment it gets personal, we can freeze. Perhaps this is because the people most intent on probing our spiritual identities on an individual level often have agendas of their own. Many aren't interested in learning or conversation but conversion and assimilation. This was something I learned firsthand.

....

BY THE TIME I ENTERED THE UNIVERSITY OF MARYLAND, College Park, I had a much better grasp of English than I'd had a few years earlier in high school. The campus was huge:

40,000 students, with space to match. Most of the dorms and classrooms, or at least the ones I went to, sat along the edges of McKeldin Mall. This was a wide-open stretch of grass the likes of which I'd never seen growing up in Tokyo, nine acres of gently sloping green crisscrossed by concrete footpaths. To my eyes, it was incredibly picturesque; it looked more like a pasture than a place of higher education. Getting around required serious footwork. During orientation week, I'd blistered my feet trekking between various sessions and seminars.

This was the mid-nineties, pre-internet. No laptops, smartphones, texting, or even email. Des'ree's "You Gotta Be" and Seal's "Kiss from a Rose" issued from seemingly every dorm room. With an associate degree and several years of work experience in Tokyo under my belt, I was significantly older than the average freshman. I'd fought to get here, studying at an extension campus at an American military base in Japan on nights and weekends, so I embraced my studies with gusto. I didn't go to many parties or sporting events. But I did make friends from all over the world. A group of British exchange students I'd been seated with during orientation took me under their wing; for the rest of the year we'd go out to eat together, hang out in each other's dorm rooms, and talk late into the night, to the point that my English started taking on a British accent.

With so much ground to cover between classes, undergrads spent large stretches of their days outdoors on foot by themselves. Religious groups took advantage of the situation, approaching new students in an attempt to convince us to join. The first few times this happened to me, I chalked it up to chance, but after a while, I started to feel as though I was being targeted. I wasn't exactly wrong. When I asked my friends, they shared similar experiences. It seemed that being propositioned by religious groups was a common rite for freshmen, and foreign students in particular. Many were far from home and family and didn't have social circles of their own. The groups often framed themselves as ways to make friends quickly. "Maybe you just look lonely," joked one of the Brits.

I vividly remember the first of my encounters. As I exited the library, which sits at the very top of McKeldin Mall, a woman strode right up to me with a big smile. "Hi, there!" she said. "Do you believe in God?" Her complexion and accent made me think she was African. She wore jeans and a sweatshirt and a backpack, like any other student, and her hair was tied back in a bundle of exquisitely tight micro braids. She was flanked by several Caucasian women, also presumably students, judging from their age and attire. The trio watched me intently as they waited for my reply.

"Uh . . ." I mumbled, after an uncomfortable pause. *Did I believe in God?* I honestly didn't know what to say. I was just trying to get to class.

The woman with the braids took a step closer. "Do you have a little time?" she pressed, her smile seemingly growing larger. "I'd love to talk more." Instinctively I took a step back. Unfazed, she began rhapsodizing about a campus Bible study group. Just as I was trying to figure out how to politely extricate myself from the conversation, a young man breezed out of the library and passed us. Watching him stride down the mall snapped me out of my shock. I apologized, a little timidly perhaps, but firmly, and marched off. The woman called out something behind me. I pretended not to hear.

Situations like this played out over and over again during my first year on campus. The evangelists who approached me were always young women, a deliberate choice, I now realize, to put me at ease. Today I'd simply ignore the intrusion altogether, or tell them to leave me alone if they proved particularly persistent. But I was a young woman who spoke English as a second language, all by herself in a foreign country, and religiously obsessed though these people might be, they were still my peers; I'd inevitably run into them on campus again. So I very much wanted to defuse rather than escalate. My hope was that they would move on and forget me.

They didn't. Over the course of my second semester, I began working on different ways to put a stop to the conversations before they began. But I quickly realized that it didn't matter. With verbal jujitsu, the faithful would twist whatever I said into an excuse for a longer interaction. "Sorry, I don't believe in God" provoked a shocked tirade about how wrong I was. "I'm not interested" didn't work, either. "I challenge your disinterest!" they'd shout as I walked past. For a while I fell back on the old standard, "I'm Buddhist," but this incited the equivalent of religious pro wrestling matches: "Tell me all about your gods and I'll tell you about my God!" At one point, I even claimed I was Jewish. No luck there, either. They just laughed and launched into the spiel anyway.

By the end of the semester, I still hadn't come up with a foolproof way of foiling religious conversations, but I started to make my peace with them. As much as these missionaries annoyed me, I had a grudging respect for their dedication. And I respected their faiths as well. I had no issues with Christians, or believers of any religions, really. The problem was one of misinterpretation. They saw my reluctance to engage as a repudiation of their spiritual identities. But my not wanting to convert had nothing to do with any distaste for their faith.

The irony was that I had, in fact, begun my academic career at a kindergarten run by Christians in Tokyo. I greatly enjoyed my time there. I don't recall anything in the way of religious education; I simply loved how they called us students their "flock of lambs."

And there was a deeper connection as well. My aunt was a Christian. She was in that old picture I mentioned finding in Chapter 1, a little girl wearing geta sandals on her feet and a big smile on her face, sitting right next to my four-year-old mother. They were cousins and lifelong friends. But I thought of her as my aunt. She lived nearby, when I was growing up, and my mother would often visit, taking me along.

I'm not sure how or when or why my aunt converted, as we never talked about religion. When I reached out to her children, my cousins, none of them knew, either. But I have some ideas. I know that she graduated from a Christian college, and that she worked for a kindergarten affiliated with it for some years after she graduated. Could she have converted back then?

When I was looking into this, I made a surprising discovery. Nearly 10 percent of the over seven hundred universities in Japan are Christian. Yet less than 1 percent of Japanese describe themselves as Christian in surveys, meaning that the vast majority of the students and faculties of these institutions do not identify as Christian. It isn't a requirement to be a Christian to enroll or work at these schools, and so a great many people of all sorts of spiritual faiths—or even no faith at all—attend them. But they do, of course, offer elective courses about Christianity. One could suppose some who were exposed to the religion in this way might become interested enough to convert. Perhaps my aunt was one of them.

My aunt loved Western things. In fact, she had dated an American before settling down with the man who would become her husband. Her relationship with a Westerner ended, but her relationship with the West only seemed to deepen. When she built her house, she chose a Western-style layout. And she outfitted several windows with stained glass, a rarity in Japanese homes. Whenever I visited, I loved looking at the vivid colors and geometric patterns, and the way they glowed when the sun passed through. My husband, when he visited with me years later, remarked that it felt like a midcentury-modern American home to him.

Her husband, my uncle, wasn't Christian for most of his life, although he converted on his deathbed, for reasons we never probed. None of her children were raised in the Christian tradition, save decking the halls with Christmas decorations every December. My aunt's faith was no secret, but none of us paid it any mind at all. It wasn't that any of us avoided the topic. It was that the very idea of talking about "faith" or "belief" never occurred to us in the first place. Japan is a place where numerous spiritual traditions coexist, and the details of what one believes in their heart of hearts is an intensely personal affair. We'd never have brought it up without her asking, and she'd never have brought it up to us, because what would have been the point? The only thing that mattered to any of us was that we loved one another. But that relationship captures how I saw Christianity: an unremarkable part of the family.

So I was shocked when I began to encounter evangelists at my university. I didn't want to become Christian, but not because of any antipathy to the faith. I didn't want to become Christian because I didn't want to limit myself. I had grown up surrounded by religious traditions and never felt pressured into declaring allegiance to any one. Why would I start now?

The last time I saw my aunt was at my wedding. She was sick, by that time, and it would be the last time she would go out by herself. She passed away soon after. Now my mother and my father have joined her.

I think about them all the time, but when I want to make things more tangible, I'll burn a stick of incense for them, because incense is the most common way for Japanese to communicate with the deceased. An outsider who saw me doing this would probably confuse this for some sort of arcane ritual—*watch the exotic Japanese worshipping her cult of ancestors*—but I don't really see things that way. Maybe it's an anniversary or holiday or special occasion; maybe I just want to have a moment.

You know how parents are. They always worry about their children, no matter how old those children get, no matter how far they might have flown from the nest. Incense is an opportunity for me to express to them that we are all doing okay, wherever they might be. For all the pain I feel, I know that the idea of my parents losing touch with my sister and me would have been even harder to bear for them. But I don't really think about it in these terms. I simply want to say hi. But, just like my grandparents were to me when I was a child, my parents are now invisible. Burning incense creates a space for me to greet them in a way that is both ritualized and casual at once.

The concept of hanshin-hangi, that mental state of half belief, half disbelief, helps explain why phrases like "ancestor worship" and "cults of ancestors" feel so lost in translation. Worship is based on faith. Faith is absolute trust in someone or something. In many Western religions, faith is a prerequisite for worship, for if you lack faith, you're just going through the motions. If one follows this logic, framing kuyo as "ancestor worship" implies that the Japanese people believe in the existence of the souls of their ancestors, which is to say, of ghosts.

But I don't know that this is the case. If you spotted a Japanese person praying in front of a stick of incense and interrupted them to ask if they believed in ghosts—please don't do this, it's a thought experiment—I suspect you'd get a deeply puzzled look. As puzzled as I was when that woman asked if I believed in God that day on campus. Because what did it really matter? Do ghosts exist? Who knows— but I can tell you we don't light sticks of incense for ghosts. We light incense, and do all sorts of kuyo, for family, for friends, for anyone whose loss deprives us—even, say, a beloved pet. Faith is a question; otherwise, why bother asking about it? But the ties to those we love are unquestionable.

Incense is a tool. To my mind, it isn't some kind of high-tech device. It's analog, timeless, less like a smartphone and more like a string telephone of the sort my little sister and I once made out of thread and paper cups. The smoldering incense is the equivalent of the cup you talk into, and the smoke rising into the air, a sort of spiritual string. I've always enjoyed watching that smoke, particularly in the moments after setting a match or lighter to the sticks, when the drab, dusty tips flush a mellow orange and the first rising tendrils of smoke caress the air like ethereal sheets of silk. Even as I know these patterns are shaped by the physics of our natural world, created by chemistry, borne on currents of wind, I can't help but think of those vapors as carrying emotions, seeking, roaming, like sacred cellular signals, until they reach the other "cup" in the spiritual world, whatever form that might take.

My burning of incense is a form of kuyo, but to be honest, I am reluctant to call it even that, because it bestows a formality that feels distancing and impersonal. The way I see it, burning incense for them isn't much different from the way I'd put on tea for some small talk when they were alive. But even if I did frame what I was doing as kuyo, one thing is for sure: It isn't religious for me at all. You might even call it a nonreligious spiritual ritual. Having said that, I wouldn't be at all surprised if a foreign observer interpreted this in religious terms. Incense arrived from China along with Buddhism, as part of the religion's rituals. This is why you'll inevitably smell it in a temple and never in a Shinto shrine.

Nobody taught me how to use incense. I guess I picked it up over the years by a kind of cultural osmosis. As a little girl I watched my parents burn it for their parents in our family's butsudan altar, communicating with their own fathers and mothers and grandparents. At temples I would see people offer incense to the Buddhist deities, placing bundles of the fragrant stuff into the cauldrons provided for that purpose in front of nearly every prayer hall. And incense plays a central role in funerals, which are often held in the Buddhist style here. As part of those ceremonies, guests approach the altar, then take turns sprinkling powdered incense into a burning censer as an offering for the departed.

And sometimes I simply enjoy its perfume. When I use it for this purpose, incense is neither religious nor kuyo. It's simply a refreshing, fun thing to do. Personally, my favorite time for burning incense is June, in the middle of Japan's legendarily damp monsoon season. I like to burn a stick in the morning, right before the rains fall, an aromatic treat to lift spirits during those weeks of overcast skies.

After its arrival with the Buddhists, incense quickly

spread from temples into households—the households of the upper crust. Close to a thousand years ago, in the eleventh century, Murasaki Shikibu, a lady-in-waiting in the imperial court of Heiankyo, put brush to paper and conjured up *The Tale of Genji*, a sprawling drama that is now widely considered to be the first modern novel. It stars a playboy known as Hikaru Genji, whose first name literally means "shining," the original beautiful young man of Japanese pop culture. His torrid affairs with a string of equally beautiful women, high-born and not, form the backbone of the story. Setting up these trysts involved cultivating a mood with subtly chosen perfumes of rare incense that telegraphed one's intentions and sophistication. To Japanese aristocrats, incense was as deeply entwined with civilization as it was with religion.

We still love incense today. We love it for its supposed purification properties—such as the incense one "bathes" in before ascending the steps to many Buddhist temples. We love it for its scents, which can relax and ease and, in so doing, perhaps even help soothe, in some small way, afflictions of body or mind. But perhaps most of all, we love incense for its spiritual flexibility. Even inside temples, there are no hard-and-fast rules. Some visitors breeze right through the clouds of incense and pray without stopping. Even among those who do tarry in the vapors, it's impossible to say how many do so out of belief, how many out of courtesy, and how many simply for fun, luxuriating in the fragrant tendrils caressing clothing and hair. Sensoji Temple, Tokyo's iconic tourist destination, possesses an enormous bronze urn, bigger than a bathtub, filled to the brim with incense ash and puffing prodigious quantities of smoke from the sheer number of offerings made by the thronging crowds. In the scrums of tourists, I often see non-Japanese who, perhaps inspired by the natives, indulge in a little incense bathing themselves. You don't have to be Japanese to appreciate the thought—or the scent. Even on holy ground such as this, the religious and secular comfortably coexist. It's what makes Japanese holy spots some of the most popular attractions in Japan.

Kuyo may have roots in Buddhism, but as widely practiced in everyday life, it isn't doctrine or dogma. It's simply a tool that gives you the freedom to hold rituals in any way you feel the most comfortable with, small or large, personal or formal. Kuyo is nondenominational spirituality. It bridges spiritualities and traditions, letting anyone incorporate the aspects they like, whether dolls or incense or whatever works for them.

But most of all, kuyo connects us to memories. The ritual, whatever form it takes, awakens precious recollections from slumber, letting us bask in their embrace once again. Perhaps the most common way in which Japanese rekindle these memories is through their butsudan, a household altar that contains memorial tablets for departed family members, and a place to burn a stick of incense to remember them. I do not possess a butsudan myself. In my typically small Tokyo home, space is at a premium, too much to spare for a piece of furniture that can range to the size of a small refrigerator.

Instead, I created a space for family photos, little visual reminders of those still in the hearts of my family. One is of my parents together. Another is of my father in his prime, wearing a dapper suit, making a speech at the lectern of a Rotary Club meeting. Next to these photos, my husband placed one of his grandfather. He had served aboard a battleship in World War II, fighting my country. But he was an early supporter of my husband's interest in Japan, even footing the bill for his first student trip there in high school. In the photo, my husband's grandfather is aboard a sailboat, azure sea beneath a cloudless sky, fishing rod in hand. He doesn't seem to have caught anything, but from the smile on his face, it looks like he's enjoying himself tremendously. He died in 1991, and I know my husband misses him, for he always remarks how much he wishes the two of us could have met. Thirty-five-odd years later, his grandfather is still in his thoughts, and this picture is a memento of that still-unspooling thread connecting the two of them.

Whenever sadness over the loss of my parents overwhelms me, it is these two photos that soothe me most, of two men who never met in life but stand together in our hearts. When I look at them, I see myself in my father, and my husband in his grandfather. They were with us then and they are within us now. Time spent with a photo can be a form of kuyo, too. This isn't ancestor worship or Confucianism or any of that. Kuyo plucks at the web of connections that link us, like fingers plucking a lute string, resonating through time and space and reminding us that, as in the old poem, no one is an island.

SOME YEARS BACK, NOT LONG AFTER MY SISTER GAVE BIRTH to her daughter, she told me she wanted to celebrate Girl's Day again.

"What happened to our old hina dolls?" I asked. "Do we still have them?"

She reported that the old boxes were there, nestled between rafters in the attic crawl space. They were dusty, she said, but intact. She suspected they hadn't been so much as touched in three decades. So it was that we decided to pull the boxes down and put up the old girls and boys.

We brought them to the living room, placed them on the floor, and sat on our knees facing the boxes. We opened the dusty lids in excitement, then froze—for, we realized, we had no idea what to do. My sister and I had never put up one of these sets before. The task had always fallen to our parents. As kids, we'd simply enjoyed the outcome. Now it was our turn.

Being older, I took the initiative, carefully shimmying off one of the tight-fitting lids from its box. Inside were layers of tissue paper, once bright and colorful, now faded to dull pastels over the decades. My mother must have packed the contents herself, protecting them from dust and jostling. As we removed the tissues, carefully as an archaeologist or paleontologist reveals their subject of study, we began to see tiny faces peeking out. In contrast to the packing material, they seemed untouched by the years. We removed them one by one, inspecting each for damage. Impressively, we found no stains, no holes in their clothing, and their porcelain faces and hands were as white as the day they'd been made, just as we remembered them from our childhoods. Beneath the dolls we excavated an instruction sheet, paper fragile from years of being unfolded and refolded, faded but readable. We opened it as carefully as we could, and consulted it like a treasure map to determine that we had nearly every piece we needed.

Even with the instructions, constructing the seven tiers of the hina display took quite a lot of trial and error. Occasionally, as we worked, we noticed some of the metal frame components were bent. From our own exertions, it was obvious that our parents had bent them in frustration at trying to get the stands set up.

"Do you think they had arguments over this?" I said to my sister.

"Probably."

My father was still alive and well at this time, and when he overheard our discussion, he rolled his eyes. We started laughing.

Once we had the stand together, the next step was draping it with its red felt cover. My sister took charge of unfurling it and using a steam iron to smooth out the folds from long decades of storage. The material was in great condition, given its age. But my sister pointed out how stained it was on the edges. When we draped it over the stands, we understood why. The stains were only on the lowest tiers, at the eye and hand level of a little girl. These were where the doll retinue's sets of tiny tea services, colorful faux sweets, intricate dowry chests, and glorious royal litters sat. That these were missing various parts confirmed that curious children had spent a lot of time exploring this part of the display.

It took an hour or two to get everything together. We gathered the family in the room, my husband, my sister's husband and daughter, and our father, whose eyes widened at seeing the set he'd last put together so many years ago assembled once again. Then we announced we were going to turn on the lanterns that flanked the emperor and empress on the top tier. We'd replaced the light bulbs but weren't sure if the old wiring would still work. With a little flourish, my sister plugged the cord into the wall outlet, and . . . Voilà! Tiny lights illuminated the royal pair once again.

My niece, not even a year old then, was too young to really appreciate the spectacle. But it seemed to transfix my father. On the lowest shelf sat a wooden plaque, inscribed with my name and date of birth in calligraphic script, made when my parents had purchased the set decades ago. It housed one of those old-fashioned windup music boxes. He picked this up and turned it over in his hands.

"We bought this set right after you were born," he said. Then he began to sing: "Akari wo tsukemasho, bonbori ni"—"Let us light the lanterns," the first line of an old song titled "Ureshii Hinamatsuri," or "Joyful Hina Festival." He wound a key on the back of the plaque and replaced it atop the stands. A soft metallic click issued from within. Then it began to play, slowly, stopping and starting mid-melody, making the perky tune sound sluggish and rusty. The mechanism was as old as I was, and it seemed it was struggling to shake off the years.

"I guess this is telling me how much time has passed," I said. We laughed as the creaky song continued to play.

....

NOW THAT MY FATHER IS GONE, I THINK ABOUT THIS MO-ment whenever I see hina dolls. It's one of many subtle triggers that developed after the loss of my parents, snares I blunder into without warning. Overhearing someone using the same ringtone I'd set for my father's incoming calls. Custard cream puffs of the sort my mother loved up to the very end. Old people on the street whose gait reminds me of one or the other of them, until my mind resolves that it isn't, couldn't be, can never be. It doesn't matter how trivial these things are: They are reminders that land with the force of a blow.

When my memories become too much to bear, I do kuyo. Sometimes I burn incense. Sometimes I just chat about them with my family and friends, remembering some good times together. It helps. It really does. Because kuyo is about memory, and memory is about love, and that will never fade. My parents are gone, but they will always be with me, a part of me.

Kuyo is about healing. Just a little. But maybe just enough.

CHAPTER 8

Radically Inclusive: Kumano

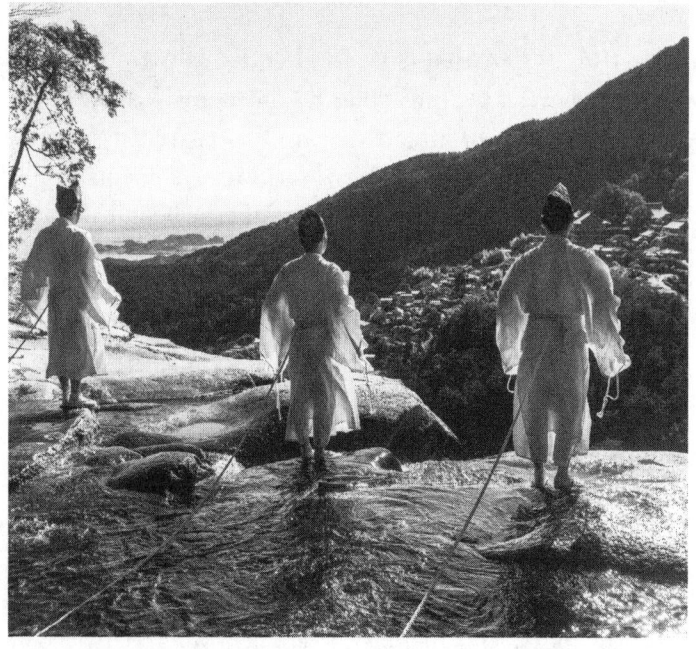

Top of Nachi Falls at Hiro Jinja shrine in Wakayama.

*Kumano is special, a holy realm where Kami and Buddhas
jostle for space.*

—Yukio Mishima

*Come as you are,
regardless of age or gender,
regardless of class high or low,
regardless of being pure or impure,
        regardless of what you believe or don't.*

—Great Avatar of Kumano

F ew Japanese profess to have a religion. But secular though our nation may seem, there remains an abiding respect for holy grounds. When we happen to be on one, the vast majority of us will pray—not necessarily out of faith but because we don't want to stand out of the crowd, and because of commonsense etiquette. But since so few Japanese go to services with any regularity, many need a helping hand in understanding what specifically they should do. In a nation where spirituality is as mixed as it is here, even natives can have a hard time differentiating between shrines and temples. Many shrines have signs with manga-like drawings illustrating how to pray there: bowing twice, clapping twice, putting palms together in prayer, and bowing once again. And it isn't at all uncommon to encounter signs at Buddhist temples reminding visitors: "This is a temple. Place your palms together quietly and pray." These two styles of prayer, one for Shinto and the other for Buddhist, are conventional wisdom, a form of common sense.

Or are they?

I was discussing the topic of prayer styles with the head priest of Kumano Hongu Taisha grand shrine, which is located in Wakayama Prefecture. It is one of Japan's most famous shrines. It's also a UNESCO World Heritage Site. There's an interesting story of how that came to be, and it upends the idea of the "right" way to pray at a shrine—at least, here in Kumano.

"Most shrines in Japan tell people that 'two bows, two claps, and one bow' is the Shinto way," head priest Ietaka Kuki said to me. He's a middle-aged man with a soft face that often breaks into a smile, as it does now.

"I get why they say it elsewhere," he continues. "It's important to have guidelines. But I believe there needs to be yawarakasa."

"Yawarakasa?" I ask. It's a word meaning "softness" or "tenderness," in literal and figurative senses.

"Yes. It is essential to prayer. Without it, I believe, people can't pray." And then Kuki tells me an interesting story.

Some years back in the first decade of the twenty-first century, the government of Wakayama, the prefecture where Kuki's shrine is located, petitioned UNESCO, the UN organization designed to promote and preserve global cultures, for World Heritage status. Nations and municipalities vie for the inclusion of their cultural sites in UNESCO's list, for prestige and public awareness, because it helps support preservation efforts and promote tourism. The region contains a celebrated network of ancient pilgrimage routes that are still widely used today. They link a great many holy sites. Kumano Hongu Taisha grand shrine is one of the biggest and most famous of them.

As part of the application process, UNESCO sent three delegates from China and European countries to investigate. They made their way around the region. But when they arrived at Kuki's shrine, the delegation came to a sudden halt in front of the gate to the prayer area.

The Japanese government had provided the delegation with an interpreter. Kuki asked her if something was wrong. It seemed one of the delegates was refusing to enter the prayer area, on the basis of his religious beliefs. Kuki gently probed: Weren't they here on official business to determine the validity of an official cultural application? He certainly wouldn't force anyone to pray. He only wanted them to see enough to make a thorough report. But nothing he said could convince the reluctant delegate. In the end, the man stayed behind while the others made their inspection. Even still, UNESCO recognized the pilgrimage routes of Kii as a World Heritage Site a few years later, in 2004.

In commemoration of that recognition, five years later UNESCO sent another delegation, larger this time, consisting of twenty or so delegates from fourteen countries. The plan was for them to experience the culture and traditions of Kumano for themselves, the better to explain them to other members back home. The group visited Kumano Hongu Taisha, of course. When they arrived, however, their interpreter told Kuki that the group wouldn't enter the prayer area. Might he simply explain the shrine from the outside, instead?

"Tell them this," Kuki said to the interpreter. "I respect that each of you has your own individual religious backgrounds. But I am hosting you as representatives of your respective nations. All I am asking is that you greet the kami in your own ways, telling them where you are from, in whatever style makes you most comfortable. Japanese traditionally bow twice, clap twice, and bow again to show respect, but you don't have to worry about that here. Do what feels right to you. Making the sign of the cross is fine.

Any custom you like is equally fine. All that matters is making a connection in a courteous way. The details do not."

"Are you sure about this, Mr. Kuki?" asked the interpreter. She had guided the delegation to many other shrines and hadn't ever heard a priest say anything like this anywhere else.

"Completely," replied Kuki. "This is the Kumano way. There are so many different countries out there, but in the end, we all want the same thing: peace. We're all in this together. If even one country feels left out, we all fall apart. That's why I want them to greet the kami themselves, and pray in their own ways."

The interpreter relayed his words to the assembled. They spontaneously applauded, something that took the interpreter by surprise, as she later told Kuki privately.

"I really thought I'd made a connection," Kuki tells me. "But guess what." He smiles again. "They all ended up praying in the Shinto style! They asked me and the interpreter to show them and we did and they all followed along. It really took me by surprise. Japanese generally just follow along when asked to do something. People abroad don't, necessarily— they make their own choices. It seems that's what happened here."

The fact that the group prayed in the Shinto way wasn't what brought him satisfaction, Kuki explained. He had no interest in converting or assimilating anyone. He simply wanted to make his visitors as comfortable as possible that they might open their hearts, and they did. That's what their praying in Shinto style at this particular moment meant: that they were willing, even for a moment, to embrace another way of thinking. And they did it because Kuki had made it clear that it wasn't about identity but about common purpose: a shared prayer for global peace, in whatever language the individuals spoke, whether linguistic or spiritual.

....

IN SO MANY FAITH TRADITIONS, BELIEF IS DEFINED IN TERMS of rejections. Where you won't go. Who you won't associate with. What you won't tolerate.

It doesn't have to be that way. Kumano testifies to that.

Kumano is the name of the region located on the tip of the Kii Peninsula, which swells out into the Pacific due south of Nara and Kyoto. If Japan's main island of Honshu were Italy, this might be called the heel of its boot. It is, or was until modern times, a remote destination reachable only through rugged terrain. If one were unaware of its history, they might be tempted to call it godforsaken.

But they would be wrong. The Kii region has long been a crossroads for pilgrims from ancient capitals of Nara and Kyoto. Far removed from the dramas and politicking of big cities, it developed an almost radical inclusiveness, welcoming to all comers, regardless of gender, class, belief, or lack thereof. The mountains of Kii are where I had my own epiphany about the nature of Japan's spirituality.

This is a place where faith blends in a way I've never seen before, anywhere else, in my home country or abroad. In the West, and particularly in immigrant cultures such as America, faith is an identity, and religious tolerance a necessity. That's a good thing, insofar as tolerance trumps intolerance. But Kumano suggests even more potential, on a personal and societal level. Simply by existing, it asks many intriguing questions:

What lies beyond tolerance?

What if you didn't have to choose a tribe?

What if different ways of thinking were worth celebrating?

What if we acknowledged that we're all in this together?

Many footpaths lead from the ancient capitals through the rugged terrain of Kii. Collectively this network is known as the Kumano Kodo, literally "the ancient Kumano trails." Ancient because they have been in use for more than a thousand years. And Kumano because all these roads lead to one place: Kumano Hongu Taisha, a grand shrine. Along the way to this Shinto spot can be found a series of key religious sites that capture virtually every "ingredient" in the "hodgepodge" of Japanese belief: Shugendo temples on Mounts Yoshino and Omine; a Buddhist temple on Mount Koya; and many other lesser-known but equally revered holy spots in between.

The trails range from gentle to rough, some carving through terrain so rugged and remote that it is called komoriku—the hidden country. Walking the hidden country feels far away but never forsaken, for those hills sing with animal life, and are dotted with tiny altars and jizo statues and markers left by pilgrims stretching back a millennium. When you walk the Kumano Kodo you may be on your own, but you will never be lonely.

Until modern times, the pilgrimage was no simple matter. The round trip from Kyoto to Kumano Hongu Taisha was many hundreds of miles, and by custom made entirely on foot. When the first pilgrims began recording their journeys, back in the tenth century, they were beset by dangers on all sides. The elements; fierce animals such as wild boar; sheer cliffs and treacherous climbs with names like Body-Breaker Slope and Abode of the Dead; bone-weariness and hunger. Locals say a yokai known as Daru haunts these paths, a creature drawn to travelers struck by starvation. Should one possess even a morsel to eat, they will be safe; if not, their continued hunger pangs and stomach groans will beckon Daru, who will pull the hapless victim into the shadows forever.

Glorious sights greeted travelers along the way. The trails wound through ancient cryptomeria cypress forests and soaring mountain peaks, over misty alpine passes and past breathtaking waterfalls. But descriptions of beauty in the records left by diarists and poets are few. Instead, their chronicles are forged in a shared language of hardship. "This route is very rough and difficult; it is impossible to describe precisely how difficult," wrote the poet Fujiwara no Teika in 1201. The Emperor Go-Shirakawa, who made the pilgrimage nearly forty times after abdicating the throne in 1158, lamented midway through one effort that he wished he could fly.

Still, they forged on. First the cultural elite, then, following their footsteps in later centuries, citizens of all walks of life from aristocrats to beggars, even outcasts and those with leprosy. As the pilgrimage grew in popularity, the trip to Kumano emerged as one of the very earliest forms of domestic tourism in Japan. But those who made this treacherous journey didn't do it for fun or leisure, or even adventure. All that was beside the point. Garbed in white, the traditional dress of a spiritual pilgrim who's left society behind, voyagers navigated toward the three grand shrines of Kumano for absolution. Yearning for forgiveness from the countless sins of previous lives, they prayed for safe passage to the Pure Land in the hereafter.

Today, the pilgrimage routes of the Kii Mountains are recognized as a UNESCO World Heritage Site, connected to the outside world by modern transport and roadways, and visited by many thousands annually. Hiking sections of the Kumano Kodo is a popular leisure pursuit for more active travelers. But even now, Kii remains far off the beaten path, removed from the hustle and bustle of major metropolises, marching to its own spiritual beat. There is much to learn from the way in which the numerous religious orders here interact with one another, collaborating and openly welcoming those of other beliefs, or even those with no beliefs, without any thought of evangelism or conversion. But this harmony was hard-won.

In fact, this organic experiment in coexistence almost came to an abrupt end during the Meiji Restoration, the late-nineteenth-century push to modernize the country. After centuries of quiet coexistence, the government compelled the nation to make a choice among its spiritual traditions, drawing hard lines between faiths and punishing any who dared cross them. It was a program of rejection, and it very nearly destroyed my entire country.

....

IN 1614, TOKUGAWA IEYASU, THE SHOGUN OF ALL JAPAN, made a fateful decision. He banned the practice of Christianity. He saw evangelism as a vehicle for European colonialism, and allegiance to this foreign god as allegiance to foreign power. So he ordered the Christian faithful rounded up and forced them to renounce their beliefs or to die. Many chose the latter. Then he sealed the nation's borders to the outside world altogether.

This status quo held for two and a half centuries. But then, in 1853, a fleet of American warships arrived unannounced in Japanese waters. The authorities long portrayed foreigners as "barbarians," but these came bearing technologies far outstripping anything known in Japan: steam engines that let them cross mighty oceans in a matter of days, and cannons that could wreak destruction with unheard-of accuracy and power. This revelation, impossible to hide from the populace at large, rocked the shogun's dynasty to its foundations. The shogunate collapsed, allowing the long-sidelined imperial family to reassert control once again. This historical moment is known as the Meiji Restoration.

Desperate to catch up with the West, Emperor Meiji and his advisers signed treaties with Western powers and devised plans to transform their feudalistic agrarian economy into a modern industrial society as quickly as possible. Among their tools were lessons gleaned from imported Western science, economics, law, politics, philosophy—and religion.

The Meiji government issued the Ordinance Distinguishing Shinto and Buddhism in 1868. This might seem an odd strategic move in the act of modernizing a country, but it was in fact deeply connected. Japan's political and intellectual leaders knew from historical experience how Christian evangelism could roil their society, and they were determined that it never happen again. So they proposed refashioning their nation's patchwork of spiritual beliefs into something better suited to withstand an onslaught of foreign proselytizing. Scholars wrote treatises on how Christianity supercharged Western politics, industry, and society, and advocated for their own faiths to take a similar role in Japan's.

There were three big problems, insofar as nationalistic imperial rulers saw it. One was that Buddhism had been the cornerstone of the Tokugawa Shogunate, a regime that they were intent on distancing themselves from. Two was the fact that Buddhism's roots were as foreign as Christianity's. And three was that Shinto, with its eight million kami, lacked a singular all-powerful deity to rally around.

Nevertheless, the government decreed that Japan, like the Western powers, would now possess a single official religion: Shinto, and Shinto alone. In order to get around the fact that it lacked a single almighty creator figure, they decreed that the emperor would now play this role. Enshrined as a living kami, he would serve as Japan's equivalent of the Western monotheists' God.

But disentangling Shugendo, Buddhism, and Shinto influences was a tall order—an impossible one, really. In the first place, there were no hard-and-fast rules delineating their holy grounds. Buddhist temples managed shrines on their properties. Shinto shrines venerated Buddhist deities right alongside kami. And Shugendo "remixed" elements of both religions into something new. We call this shinbutsu shugo, which literally means "Shinto-Buddhist fusion." In some places, the fusion was so thorough that it birthed entirely new, homegrown deities that bridged both faith systems: Gongen, or avatars, like Zao Daigongen, whose epic statues I visited at Kinpusenji temple in Yoshino.

With the bureaucratic equivalent of a snap of the fingers, the authorities tried to reverse centuries of history. Temples were ordered to remove Shinto imagery, and shrines, their Buddhist imagery. Avatars were banned. Shugendo and Buddhist monks were forbidden from participating with shrines in any capacity, unless they renounced their orders and converted to Shinto.

Chaos ensued.

Today, we call it haibutsu kishaku, which is written with characters meaning "the elimination of Buddhism." It was a radical populist movement that wasn't explicitly supported by the government but was certainly fueled by its policies and rhetoric. It eventually resulted in the outright destruction of some forty thousand temples. Many other parishes effectively disappeared when their monks quit, out of despondency or fear, or both.

When it came to Shugendo, the government took an even harder line, banning its practice outright in 1872. There was simply no way to untangle the threads of spiritual influences that intertwined in the fabric of its tradition. Instead, they forced the yamabushi, then some 170,000 strong, to make an impossible decision: Declare themselves purely Shinto or Buddhist. Kinpusenji, that Shugendo epicenter with the glorious effigies of the avatar Zao Daigongen, chose the former path. The yamabushi closed a pair of enormous wooden doors to hide the titanic statues from public view, then placed a mirror in front of the altar to make it a Shinto shrine. The Great Avatar of Zao wouldn't reemerge from the shadows until freedom of religion was restored by constitutional decree in 1947, seventy-five years later. The span of a human lifetime.

Even though Japanese people have been free to practice whatever beliefs they see fit since then, the legacy of the anti-Buddhist campaign can still be seen today, in ways large and small. Scars on stone monuments where Buddhist sanskrit lettering was chiseled away. Sad little jizo statues with their heads missing, lopped off in those crusades of a century or more ago. More than once I have encountered a moss-covered staircase of stone in the forest, once leading to a temple, now leading nowhere.

And then there are absences you don't even realize are there, until you're confronted with them. Some years back, I spent quite a bit of time in the archives of a major Asian art museum in the United States conducting research for a book. Their holdings naturally included a great many religious works, and as I moved from place to place behind the scenes, I would inevitably pass gorgeous statuary being restored or prepared for display.

One struck me in particular: a desktop-size wooden

statue of Aizen Myo'o, a Buddhist embodiment of righteous anger. This is a ferocious-looking deity with crimson skin. Its head is topped by a roaring lion. Flaming hair frames a scowling face. And six arms clutch esoteric weaponry for spiritual battles.

This tiny but fierce portrayal, no more than a foot tall, was very old. Its surface had dulled to ashen tones, its colors muted by centuries of dust and soot from fire rituals and incense. The statue stirred a great deal of complicated feelings in me. Who had once venerated it? And what was it doing here, oceans away from home in a land unknown to its creators, moved from a bustling temple to this unremarkable hallway, its fluorescent lighting, bare walls, and drab carpet as close a metaphor for purgatory as one might imagine?

I'm no historian, but it was obvious this statue wasn't the kind of thing someone would simply decide to let go. That's when it dawned on me: It had probably been sold off in the midst of that anti-Buddhist chaos. I don't mean to cast any aspersions here. I knew the curators were doing their utmost to care for this priceless piece of my nation's heritage, and for that I was grateful. When my country's leaders began destroying our Buddhist heritage, foreign collectors stepped in to rescue many precious pieces of art. Still, knowing the little statue had been taken from its home, from those who loved and cherished it in the first place, made me deeply sad as well. Was its presence here a ripple effect of that sad legacy, a quiet testament to the hidden costs of the Meiji aristocrats' misguided plan? Whatever the case, I knew this statue had been lucky to survive the purge. Many others did not.

So it was that twelve centuries after Buddhism's triumph in Japan, it and Shugendo were pushed to the brink of extinction—all in the name of so-called progress, civilization, and enlightenment. But this was no victory for Shinto. In fact, the mayhem was only beginning. As the forcible streamlining of spirituality in Japan forged full steam ahead, the authorities compelled local shrines to merge with larger ones, the better to keep an eye on parishioners. Then they made this reorganization official law in 1906. At the time, there was something like two hundred thousand Shinto shrines in all of Japan. Over the next eight years, a third of them would be effectively wiped out.

This was framed as progress. But we know what really happened. The choosing of sides and drawing of lines had terrible consequences. Forcing Shinto into the role of national religion paved the way for the nationalism, authoritarianism, and imperialism of the early twentieth century: suffering and sorrow on a global scale. But the effects of the government's decision first played out locally, in ways few could have anticipated, in places unexpected.

In that great Meiji rush to modernization, the government commanded Kumano to shut down about 80 percent of its shrines, the better to consolidate control over a select few. Then it doubled down by ordering the harvesting of the groves in which they had stood, as lumber was then one of Japan's most precious resources. Entire old-growth forests disappeared, milled into boards for export to rapidly expanding cities. The hills lost their ancient natural protection against the elements. In 1889, torrential rains caused mudslides. The mudslides created a series of natural dams up in the mountains. As the rain continued, they burst. A deluge of water and debris washed over Kumano, killing more than two hundred residents and washing the grand shrine away. This was but a taste of the "progress" that would soon rack Japan, and then the region, and then the world.

AS I WRITE THIS HISTORY, STEEPING MYSELF IN A PARTICU-larly dark period for my people, memories of my own dark times inevitably bubble to the surface.

There was a point in my life where I tried to define myself by rejecting Japan. The reckoning began a few years out of junior college, when I quit my job. This might not sound like much of a big deal today, but it certainly was in Japan of the early nineties. I'd been working full-time only for a few years, and this sort of life change was pretty much unheard of. Once you joined a company, you were expected to work there for life. Unless you were a woman. In that case, you were expected to work until you married, at which point you'd be heavily encouraged to quit so that you could focus on being a full-time housewife and mother. Society euphemistically called this kotobuki-taisha, which meant "joyful retirement," but it didn't sound particularly joyful to me. I'd read American women describing their workplaces as having a glass ceiling. Japan's weren't even transparent.

My time as an exchange student had left a deep impression on me, and in the years since, I'd developed an interest in global politics. When I took a job, I expected I'd need to pay my dues; I never complained when I was directed to serve tea to executives and guests. But after a while, I noticed that only female employees were being asked to do it. And that we stayed in our junior positions, while the young men who'd joined at the same time as us were fast-tracked for promotions.

I'd spent junior and senior high in all-girls schools, and graduated from a women's college. This bubble isolated me from the inequalities of society at large. In college, I'd dreamed about working abroad. In fact, I'd specifically chosen this company because it was multinational, with branch offices all over the globe. I dreamed of transferring to one of those branches someday, learning more about the world, perhaps even spending my career overseas.

Only after I'd signed on did I learn the company had an unspoken policy of never transferring women to foreign offices. I'd learned this when I asked a manager about working abroad.

"We've found that girls are happiest here at headquarters," he replied. *Girls*. He didn't even mean it in a condescending way. He was perfectly earnest, even solicitous, as though he were doing us a favor. Somehow that made it even worse.

This was a major, well-respected company. It was my first time confronting the reality of sexism in my society— and a sexism so entrenched that I had no hopes of overcoming it. Over the months, frustration fermented into quiet anger. If my country was going to treat women this way, I would leave. I didn't even care if I ever came back.

I began attending night classes at an American airbase on the outskirts of Tokyo, then I returned to America, where I enrolled for a four-year university degree. Then I went on to get my master's. I moved from my suburban Maryland college campus to the city of Washington, DC. These were fruitful, exciting years. I went to many places and met many people, including the American who would eventually become my husband.

At first I'd thrown myself into absorbing American ways, deliberately casting what I thought of as "Japanese things" aside. I strove to live and interact with Americans as a native would, rewiring my identity to mirror what I saw reflected by the natives around me. It worked for a while, but soon I began noticing cracks in my new facade. The fundamental problem was, I wasn't American. Whenever I suppressed my Japanese instincts and tried to compete with

Americans, I felt as though I was playing a sport with one arm tied behind my back. A part of this was linguistic, in the sense that I wasn't a native speaker. But a bigger part was cultural. I was acting American, but deep down I still thought, and felt, Japanese.

The more time I spent in America trying to fit in, the more I had to admit I found myself missing Japan. I didn't miss the chauvinism, of course. But I missed my family—there were no video meeting apps back then, and long-distance phone calls were expensive and infrequent. And there was something more. I'd left Japan to avoid being hammered down into what society expected of a woman. Now I was hammering myself down, into what I imagined American society expected of me.

I'd grown up in Japan, spent two decades of my life there. This bedrock wasn't something I could chisel away. There were great things about the way Americans lived and dreamed, how they stood up for themselves, how they strove for equality; even if they didn't always succeed, the fact that they tried resonated deeply with me. But there were other aspects that rubbed me the wrong way.

For instance, I noticed a tendency toward defining oneself through negatives. What someone *wasn't*, or what they didn't like, whether it was a food or a musical artist or politician or whatever, took on an outsize importance. Sometimes it veered into outright challenge—*What, you* like *that* (fill in the blank)?

And that same assertiveness that made Americans so American often made me feel as though I was getting steamrolled. If you wanted to make your position understood, you had to be ready to lock horns. If Japanese communication was like Aikido, the martial art in which opponents spar without using overt force, then American discourse felt more like boxing. I often felt like I was going into conversations with my dukes up.

Mind you, it wasn't that I saw the Japanese way as *better*. I'd left for a reason, a valid one that still deeply upset me. The problem was that suppressing my Japanese side wasn't working. Looking back, I was struggling to devise a way to bridge the worlds within me, to pick and choose the parts that served me well and build something new, to find a new equilibrium based on the best of both. Years later, I would apply this same paradigm to my spiritual thinking. Now I realize that journey began here. Balance isn't about crushing differences but embracing them.

To put it in musical terms, it's like a choir, an ensemble of different voices, sometimes singing in unison, sometimes stepping up for solos. The tenors aren't superior to the sopranos, or the altos to the bass. Each plays an important role in the harmony. There are no sides in a choir, only parts. You start choosing sides in a choir, and everything falls apart.

WHEN I RETURNED TO JAPAN IN MY EARLY THIRTIES, IT WAS not in the spirit of repudiation; it was a personal evolution. Rejecting Japan hadn't worked out for me, so regardless of my frustrations, I knew that rejecting America wouldn't work, either. How could I? By this time I had married an American.

My husband and I launched a translation business, and so I could live and work in Japan on my own terms. So went the next decade. I took pride in all this, in our entrepreneurship, in our successes and ability to endure the many struggles that come with running a company.

Living in Japan, I found myself slipping back into cultural traditions, as easily as I might slip into a comfortable favorite sweater at the first cold snap. Reaching for the thick rope to ring the jangly bells at Shinto shrines. Hiking old mountain paths that Shugendo yamabushi once walked. Sweeping leaves and weeds from my family's graves. Saying a little prayer whenever I passed a roadside jizo statue.

But this time I found myself unsatisfied with simply doing. I wanted to know more. Like a sweater, cultures are woven from threads. Where did the threads I was following come from? How were they woven? Where might they lead?

I lost my mother in 2008, just a few years before I turned forty. That sparked the journey I've been chronicling in the pages of this book. One of the first places I sought out was Kumano. It came up again and again in my studies, in my readings, in texts and histories and stories ancient and modern.

One of the things that drew me here was that, unlike so many other holy spots in Japan, Kumano was always open to everyone—including women. Echoing the sexism of male-dominated society, both Shinto and Buddhism viewed us as impure, tainted by our association with blood. Mount Fuji was off-limits to women until 1872. And I've written about my frustration at not being able to climb the Shugendo mountain of Sanjogatake. But not Kumano. Never Kumano. Its salvation has always been open to all comers.

Unlike the pilgrims of old, I traveled to Kumano by train. And I navigated among its sites through the modern contrivance of a rental car. I made my first stop the site of the old Kumano Hongu Taisha grand shrine, just after sunrise on a rainy spring morning.

Its entrance was framed by the largest tori'i gate I had ever seen—in fact, at 108 feet tall, the largest tori'i in all of Japan, so large it towers over the nearby cryptomeria cypress grove. The path leading through the gate cut through rice paddies. In another month they would sport the beginnings of their emerald coats, bundles of tiny rice shoots questing out from the muck in orderly rows. But that day the paddies were filled with mud, waiting patiently for the planting to come.

As I passed between the pillars of the gate, the air was thick with the resinous scent of cryptomeria cypress. Nobody was around, save the birds; the only sound was the chirping of crickets and the babbling of the Kumano River. Countless pilgrims had set out for this destination, from homes in distant realms. So many made the journey here that it gave rise to a famed saying: "like a line of ants, making its way to Kumano." Now I, too, was an ant, dwarfed by the tori'i and soaring cypress, making my way to the same destination.

I wanted to walk the ground pilgrims had walked, to see what they had seen. But I knew the grand shrine wasn't there anymore. Inside the grove beyond that massive tori'i gate, where the shrine once stood, now lies an open field, with only a series of stone monuments marking the spot where so many had once come seeking solace, rejuvenation, rebirth—or simply to say their thanks.

Kumano is home to a cluster of holy sites: There's Kumano Hongu Taisha grand shrine, of course, but also Kumano Hayatama Taisha, and Kumano Nachi Taisha, which is famed for its beautiful waterfall, Nachi Falls. The falls are treated as their own shrine within the larger shrine complex. Hiro Jinja, whose name translates into "shrine of the flying waterfall," lay up in the mountains, about half an hour by car from the grove of the original grand shrine. That is where I headed next.

The shrine of the flying waterfall's name is no exaggeration. It sits at the base of a sheer rock face that soars 436 feet into the sky. From the precipice far above, the Nachi River plunges and transforms into a waterfall that empties into a jumble of massive boulders. A series of stone stairs, worn smooth by centuries of footsteps, leads to the base of the waterfall. On the day I visited, the steps were slick from rain, and I needed to pick my way down them carefully so as not to slip and fall.

At the bottom of the stairs stood a shrine with several buildings and a tori'i gate. This gate was smaller than the one I had passed through back in town, but impressive nonetheless, for it framed Nachi Falls like a giant view-finder. The mist thrown up by endlessly cascading water—up to a ton a minute at peak times, I was told—nourished groves of cypress and a glorious tangle of mosses and vines that carpeted the cliff face. Fed by the rains, the waterfall literally roared. I could feel the sound as it ricocheted off the stone and washed over my body in waves, like a drum, like a heartbeat. I bathed in it.

This is a dragon, I thought.

The Japanese language is written with three different syllabaries. Two are native, phonetic scripts. The other is adapted from Chinese, and more symbolic. We call those characters kanji. You can "dissect" the components of them to discern the subtleties of their meanings, in a sort of visual analogue to the Latin roots of Romance languages. It's a lot of fun to do, when you know the basics. For instance, the kanji character for "waterfall" looks like this.

瀧

Look closely. The three dashes at the far left are a visual shorthand for splashing water. And the rest means "dragon." You can almost make out a head and tail at the right, a remnant of when characters like this were drawn as more literal pictograms, millennia ago. I love this visual aspect of my language, because it speaks in ways different from phonetic text like our domestic scripts, or the Western alphabet. When you look with the right eyes, it sings. Or roars.

In the West, dragons are dangerous monsters. The Bible treats "dragon" as a synonym for villainy. They are stereotypical antagonists in fairy tales and fantasy, like the venal Smaug, hoarder of treasure in *The Hobbit*. But in Asia, dragons are different. We imagine them as large, serpentine creatures with clawed feet who can fly into the sky, conjuring clouds and storms and wind. To us, dragons dwell not in the depths but in the heavens, icons of luck and fortune and powers beyond imagination. But most of all, they symbolize water. Dragons are rain-bringers, which means they are life-bringers.

At Nachi Taisha the waterfall is freighted with even more meaning. It is more than just a waterfall: It is a symbol of a kami. This shrine had no prayer hall; instead, the tori'i gate framed the falls. At the top of the precipice, high above, I could see a shimenawa, the braided rope used to delineate sacred places in Shinto, stretched right over where the waters made their dramatic plunge. Shimenawa, being exposed to the elements, need to be renewed regularly, and this one was particularly exposed, by the roaring mists and winds from the water rushing endlessly below. *How on earth do they change that?* I wondered. Whatever the case, it was clear that the cliff and basin and everything surrounding it were holy ground. When you prayed here, you prayed to the falls. And thanks to the rainy weather, I had them pretty much to myself today.

I stood there contemplating the waterfall for quite some time. The longer I watched, the more details began to emerge. What at first looked like a continuous flow of water was, in fact, composed of countless individual falling streamlets, each like a miniature of the whole unto themselves. To my eyes these looked like smaller dragons, their bodies twisting and changing in shape and size as they swooped down the cliff face.

And then I caught something out of the corner of my eye: The terrain around the falls seemed to be swelling and contracting. Was it some optical trick, from having shifted my gaze from the vertical motion to the immobile background? Whatever it was, it looked like a rhythmic rise and drop, as though the stone and soil were breathing. This was no longer a static feature of terrain but a living thing, as full of vigor as the enormous cypress that flanked the falls. And was it just me, or had the falls actually grown?

They had. The flow had definitely increased, widening, ropes of water joining into a thick curtain that obscured the wall behind and fanned over the rocks below. Heavier rain must have been on the way, the swell of the falls a sign it was already falling farther upstream. By this point a fog had begun to gather, shrouding the precipice above in thick cloud. Soon the water appeared to be issuing straight out of the sky, as though the handiwork of a dragon or kami, or both.

I'd come here to Kumano because I was interested, but also because I was frustrated. I had spent years studying Japanese history, folklore, culture, traditions, and religion. I'd passed my Shinto Cultural Examinations. I had been to so many holy spots and spoken to many spiritual leaders. Yet still I struggled to articulate the lessons I'd internalized.

My interest in Japanese spirituality wasn't some kind of hobby. I had come to realize that it was a quiet force that had guided me through many of my life choices. I spent most of my twenties living outside of Japan, interacting with people of all sorts of ethnic and religious backgrounds. I studied for my master's degree in America and the Middle East. And for many years after that, I made a living running a localization company, translating all sorts of Japanese content for consumers around the globe. My passion was building bridges between my country and the world. Linguistically, perhaps, I'd succeeded. Those countless video games and comic books, the toys and entertainment of all kinds I'd worked on—they had helped stoke an interest in Japan that seemed to be growing by the day. But spiritually? That was another matter.

I longed to explain how we saw the world. How we grow up surrounded by many religions, yet rarely declare allegiance to any particular one. How millennia of spiritual traditions have been so woven into the fabric of modern, daily life that even we don't really notice them. How we mix and match and choose among those traditions without feeling the need to ask permission, to defend or declare our decision.

The dramatic assertiveness of Western faithful can overwhelm Japanese unaccustomed to wearing their spiritual identities on their sleeves. Our failure, our inability, to engage on the same terms makes us seem indecisive, even devoid of faith, to outsiders. I'd experienced this myself, on that homestay in Indiana, all those years ago. But I quickly learned it wasn't simply some small-town thing. The idea that faith demanded declarations and renunciations was pervasive at all levels of Western society, but it was particularly pronounced in America. I noted how many foreign reports portrayed Japan as being in a spiritual crisis. The mass media repeatedly framed my country as among the world's least religious countries, or "nonreligious," of our religious traditions being in "irreversible decline," or even that we were a nation of atheists.

The reporters and pollsters were obviously asking the

wrong questions—they had to be, with the number of Shinto shrines and Buddhist temples in my country. They interpreted our reluctance to declare allegiance to any one faith as a lack of belief, as an empty void. For in the West, emptiness is a synonym for desolation, vacuity, loss. But to us, emptiness represents potential. Emptiness accommodates rather than excludes, fertilizing a spirituality rooted not in dogma or doctrine but in sentiments, in emotions, in feelings. Once I asked a Shinto priest what he imagined when he thought of the kami. "They have no form," he had said. "They're like a place in your heart."

When I was in America in that high school exchange program, I'd had the opportunity to visit Niagara Falls. I'd never seen anything like it. Niagara's Horseshoe Falls is only about a third the height of Nachi Falls but is many, many times wider—something like 2,500 feet across. The sheer volume of water cascading over the gracefully curved edge, the ceaseless roar, the spray—the spectacle sent a shiver of joy down my spine, even as a seventeen-year-old. This was the kind of thing that reminded you of your place in the universe, in a good way. A testament to the power of nature, the nature that created us, and sustained us, and to which we'd return in the end of it all. The falls were a miracle.

Now, decades later, I was in Kumano, gazing up at another waterfall, yet feeling that same sense of awe and gratitude. The only difference between the two being that one was a Shinto shrine, and the other was a tourist attraction. Did that mean what I felt at Nachi Falls was religious, and what I felt at Horseshoe Falls was not? That couldn't be right.

"Magnificent, isn't it?" came a voice from behind, raised just enough so that I could hear it over the roaring water.

I turned to find a man, tall, middle-aged. He was dressed

in the daily wear of a Shinto priest, a thin white robe and billowy hakama trousers in pale blue.

"Looks like you and the falls had a lot to say to each other," he said with a smile.

I looked at my watch. I was shocked to realize I'd been standing there for two and half hours. He must have been wondering what I was doing standing out there in the drizzle and fog. I shook my head and laughed. I told him it was hard to break away from something so beautiful.

"We get many visitors here every day," he said. "And each and every one of them gets something from the falls. Maybe it's an idea. Maybe it's just a feeling. Whatever it is, it means something."

When I mentioned that I'd only dropped by on my way to the grand shrine, the priest beckoned me over to the office, where he offered me a printed map of the area. He encouraged me to take my time and explore. "You never know what you'll find."

It was from that map that I learned Nachi Taisha grand shrine sat next to a Buddhist temple, Seiganto-ji. And then, as I finally turned to leave the falls, I noticed a small wooden building, just behind the shrine's offices. Curiosity got the better of me and I went over. It was small, perhaps only six feet square, constructed of beautifully joined unpainted timber. Its front doors, opened like a pair of shutters, were covered top to bottom in wooden talismans with kanji characters painted in precise calligraphy. Inside the doors, I could see an octagonal firepit, now silent. And behind it was a statue, ancient and worn, but meticulously maintained. It was of En the Ascetic, the founder of Shugendo.

This was a Shugendo prayer hall, maintained by Shinto priests, in the shadow of a Buddhist temple just up the hill. A mixture of foreign and domestic traditions, set to the soundtrack of roaring waters on a stage of soaring evergreens.

This place wasn't dedicated to Shinto, or Buddhism, or Shugendo specifically. It was much bigger than that. It has a deeper meaning no matter where you are from—Kumano, or New York, or anywhere else. Japan's spiritual traditions may be cultural, but they're based in something all of us can share, because all of us came from it: the world that created us. When nature shows us its beauty, it is more than just a pretty sight. The natural world is a reminder of everything that created us, and can unmake us, and that supports us. That is something deserving of our respect and gratitude. That is the stage against which every single drama of our lives plays out, birth and death, joy and sorrow, failure and triumph.

That is what I got from my "conversation" with the falls.

Much later, I would come across a book written by the yamabushi Riten Tanaka, former head priest of Kinpusenji Temple. "When foreigners see Japanese people praying to the falls at Nachi, they often ask what we are praying to," he wrote. "They wonder if we are worshiping the water itself, and if that's the case, how far do we go—are we worshiping the river? All the way to the sea into which it flows? But we aren't actually worshiping the water itself. The power of that water is the power of nature, and *that* is the divine, that something greater than ourselves."

You never know what you'll find.

··

FROM HIRO JINJA, I MADE MY WAY DOWN THE MOUNTAIN, past the floodplain where the old grand shrine once stood, and to the new Kumano Hongu Taisha. It sits on higher ground, atop a series of stone staircases. Part of the reason for building it atop higher ground was pragmatic. But an equal or even greater reason was spiritual.

"They took the flood as a sign from the kami," head priest Kuki wrote in a history of the area. "Showing anger, telling us to go back to our origins. We leave the former shrine grounds primitive, as they were before even the original shrine was built, as a reminder: we co-exist with nature."

I prepared to pray in the Shinto style—two bows, two claps, one bow—for this was a Shinto shrine, after all. But then a Buddhist monk strode up next to me, in full robes, and began chanting sutras with his rosary in hand.

This wasn't something you'd normally expect to see at a shrine. It wasn't that Buddhists were excluded from visiting shrines—far from it. But you generally didn't see anyone praying in the Buddhist style at them, let alone ordained monks.

It was obvious that things were different here, that people here felt free to pray in whatever style suited them. Over the course of my trip, I'd return both to Nachi Falls and the grand shrine several times. I saw a huge variety of people praying and paying respects in their own ways. Shinto and Buddhist devout. New Agers. Foreigners from all over the world, and dressed in all sorts of ways, from formal clothing to hiking gear.

Once, I even saw a woman offering up a flamenco dance. Early one morning I spotted her as I approached the grand shrine just after dawn. Nobody was around save us. She was middle-aged and Japanese, and had placed a portable stereo on the stone steps. I watched her twirling in the morning light, the crimson of her dress flickering like flames against the earthtones of the shrine's stone-and-wood structure. I didn't get the sense she was a pro, just someone who loved dancing. I'd never seen anything like this at a shrine or any other holy spot, for that matter. I watched in fascination as the song played out.

Kumano was that sort of place. So remote and removed from society, even today, that simply arriving felt like an achievement. Kumano wasn't somewhere you stumbled upon: You had to commit to going there. And in return for that commitment, it welcomed you, whoever you were, whatever you were. To step into Kumano was to step into yourself. And who was to say a flamenco dance, given with one's full heart, was any more or less worthy than a formal Shinto offering? Those were conventions dreamed up by humans, after all. Here was a place you could bare your heart to the kami, and know they would understand, whoever you are, whatever you believed.

I should note here that I don't mean to give the impression that *anything* goes at Kumano. This was an unusual case. Shrines, all shrines, are holy sites and should be approached with restraint and respect. As a foreign visitor you don't need to master any formal etiquette or customs, but you can use a simple question to guide your behavior there, or at any other holy spot in Japan: *Would I do this at a church, a synagogue, or a mosque in my home country?* And if the answer is no, then you shouldn't do it at a shrine or temple, either. I am thrilled by the interest visitors from abroad have in my country's spiritual traditions and places. But some visitors seem to treat Japan's holy grounds as theme parks, waltzing around in shorts and flip-flops, eating in the sanctuary, or using it as a backdrop for social media or streaming businesses. Again: *Would you do this on holy ground in your own country?* Even the flamenco dancer knew to limit her performance to the early hours when few would be around, and kept the volume of her music to a reasonable level. This wasn't about showing off or having fun; it was about showing respect in a uniquely personal way.

Unique, because each of the kami is different. Each plays a different role. Some are, to put it in human terms, flashier than others. Some are avatars for things we would really rather avoid. There are, for instance, kami of plague, famine, and poverty. This doesn't mean we worship or praise them. But we can't reject them. No matter how much we fear these things, or wish that we didn't have to deal with them, it is a fact that we do. And we must recognize that fact to deal with them, in whatever human ways we can. That is what kami are all about. This is why *eight million* isn't intended literally. It is poetic shorthand for the infinite. There is always room for more.

And you don't have to declare yourself a Shinto believer to feel them. You can feel them in that shiver down your spine when you look at something beautiful. Shrines are places, but they don't have to be. Like the kami themselves, they can be in your heart. These days, Japan's pop culture is hugely popular around the world. Anime and manga lead the way, but games, music, and literature play big parts, too. Perhaps because of this exposure to so much content made in Japan, I've noticed a growing interest in Japanese spirituality as well.

Whenever the topic comes up in English, online or in conversation, I often encounter the word *Shintoism*. I have even heard foreign people claim to be Shintoist. Their hunger for knowledge fascinates me, and their desire to be included warms my heart. But *Shintoism* sounds incredibly strange to my native ears.

The word *Shintoism* dates back to those first years after Japan's opening to the West, as foreign observers and local leaders scrambled to come up with a way to describe our patchwork of traditional beliefs. The problem is that an "-ism" misses the entire point of Shinto. An "-ism" is an ideology. An "-ism" is an identity. An "-ism" draws a boundary that separates itself from other things. It was coined, I think, out of insecurity—that Shinto somehow needs an "-ism" to "compete" with organized religions, where faith hinges on a contract with an almighty god. But it can also breed misunderstandings. Those who see Shinto as an "-ism" often assume that there is some hierarchy among the eight million kami, with, for instance, Amaterasu the Sun Goddess atop it all. But it doesn't work that way.

Perhaps my resistance comes from my knowledge that Japan actually did create a hierarchy, once, back in Meiji, but it failed. More than failed. It almost destroyed us. Shinto is described as a religion, but it's really, in very literal terms, a way—the Way of the Kami. And ways aren't destinations. They are paths for journeys, and can start, stop, pick up where we left off—it's all up to us.

IN DECEMBER OF 2022, I RETURNED TO HIRO JINJA AND NA-chi Falls. This time, it was a beautiful day, without a cloud in the sky. But once again, I couldn't see the waterfall. The reason being that I was standing on top of it, on its precipice, 436 feet above the shrine.

Let me set the stage. Above the falls, you'll recall, at the very top where the water begins its dramatic cascade, is strung a shimenawa. This braided rope is changed twice a year, in a special ceremony that is off-limits to the public. A few months back, I'd asked a friend of mine, who happens to be friends with several Shinto priests in Kumano, how they changed it. He offered to put me in touch with them.

While anyone can watch the priests work from the base of the falls, the swapping of the shimenawa is a religious ceremony, and one conducted in a precariously high place. Outsiders generally aren't allowed to accompany the priests to the top of the falls. But when I explained to the priests that I was writing a book—this book—they made an exception.

So it was that I found myself here, atop the falls, giving me the dizzying perspective of seeing the shimenawa up close, and from the opposite side. My vantage point was on a rocky bank of the Nachi River, which here runs wide and shallow, its flow gentle, giving little hint of the energies that will be unleashed once it makes that eternal leap over the edge.

A decade had passed since my "conversation" with the falls, down at the bottom. Now here I was, at the very top. *Moving up in the world*, I chuckled to myself, partly to hide my terror. This was, without a doubt, the highest place upon which I had ever stood. I'd flown much higher in jets, of course. Or looked out from higher vantages in skyscrapers. But those were rooms, more or less, experiences mediated by walls and glass and railings. There was no mediation here. There was nothing between me and the great beyond save air. And gravity.

Straight ahead—I couldn't bring myself to look down—I could see a valley stretching into the distance, cut over eons into the terrain by the relentless flow of this very water. Tucked into that valley were the Buddhist temple, Seiganto-ji, side by side with Kumano Nachi Taisha, nary a fence between them: spiritual siblings cheek to cheek in a cradle of stone.

That complex is where I had begun the climb up. Before I departed, a Shinto priest had swished an onusa, a wand of paper streamers, over my head and recited a little prayer. This was a ritual to spiritually purify those who would enter holy ground. Which this entire mountain was.

I began to climb a steep and narrow trail cut through cedars, towering and aromatic. But I also picked up the scent of something you'd normally never encounter at a Shinto shrine: incense, wafting up from a service at the temple. It was another reminder that the Japanese kami and Buddhist hotoke live together here in Kumano, a tradition of quiet coexistence that has been carefully curated since ancient times, handed down generation to generation, tended like the embers of a sacred flame.

It took about an hour to work my way up to the top of the falls, switchbacking through the cedars. Eventually, I reached a sign proclaiming the trail beyond off-limits to all but the priests and those they allowed to accompany them on their rituals. Beyond it the path forked to a bank of the Nachi River, which on this day looked more like a stream, perhaps twenty feet wide but only a few inches deep, with steep banks of earth exposing the gnarled roots of ancient trees. I picked my way downstream, keeping to the edge, atop wobbly rocks and slick mud, using the roots for balance. A thick canopy of leaves stretched above, making it feel as though I were walking down a tunnel. When I rounded the last bend, I was dazzled by blazing light—the opening where the river dropped off into the falls. At the precipice had already gathered a small group of priests and assistants, absorbed in preparations for their ritual, their bodies silhouetted by the morning sun.

Few get to experience this bird's-eye view of Kumano, and I wanted to savor it for as long as I was able. I settled into a comfortable spot, a few feet from the edge, where I could put a solid wall of rock behind me for physical—and, let's be honest, emotional—support. From this perch I could just make out the red spire of Seiganto-ji's three-storied pagoda. Far beyond it lay the sea, framed between gentle mountain slopes like an ukiyo-e woodblock print. And even farther beyond stretched the sky, deep cerulean, cloudless and pure.

Then there was the shimenawa. It was a sturdy white rope strung directly above the falls, ends tied to trees on either side of the river. A shimenawa is a Shinto icon, but it's also a visual code: *This place is special. This place is awe-inspiring. This place is worthy of respect.* Tying one above the falls is a sign of respect for the waters, but it's also a sign of respect for the earth itself, the powers and forces beyond our control. Normally, these forces are invisible; here, in the form of a shallow stream that transforms into a roaring waterfall, we can see that power with our own eyes. The sense of awe we feel at these natural forces is what drew seekers, from ancient times to the present day.

The shimenawa is replaced once in winter and once in summer. This was December, making the ceremony doubly important as it also marked the new year to come, a time of reflection and renewal. From the bottom of the falls, the rope looked threadlike, dwarfed by the massive terrain. Up close, I realized what a misperception this was. It wasn't as thick as some shimenawa I'd seen, but it was sturdy and long. Later, I would be told it stretched eighty-five feet from end to end.

The priests, their waists tied with lifelines held by groups of men farther upstream, wrestled with the rope. Its weight shifted unpredictably, as though it were a living thing. The waters were only about ankle deep, but this was winter, and the men worked in thin white robes and straw sandals. But never did I hear anyone complain, or see anyone shiver. For the better part of an hour they continued hefting the rope, adjusting it, dropping it, and rehanging until it was just right.

Once they were satisfied with the position of the shimenawa, the priests strode under it and to the very edge of the falls. Standing in a row on the precipice, they bowed in unison to the expanse before them, the winter sun blazing far above, their own shrine and Seiganto-ji temple far below, and the mountains and sea beyond. No words were spoken, no prayers read, for prayers are human speech, and this ritual wasn't for us. It was for the falls, and the mountains and skies and everything beyond.

The sun gave the robes and the shimenawa's streamers an incandescent glow; the surface of the river glistened like unseen hands were scattering jewels. Even the evergreen needles seemed to take on a resinous glow. Water was the only sound, the sound of water surging off the cliff, the sound of water crashing far below.

Even a happy year's end can be a bittersweet time, filled with memories of all that we've done, tinted with the knowledge that another measure of our lives has slipped into memory. But I found myself swelling with gratitude. Gratitude for having made it through another year. Gratitude for having met new people and having gone to new places. The moment was a reminder that a year, that construct of human time, wasn't really an end at all but the continuation of an ongoing journey. Instinctively, I found myself bowing along with the priests, thanking the kami, thanking nature, for making this moment happen.

As the assembled began packing up for the trek back down into the valley, I saw one of the priests taking a breather at the edge of the cliff. He had shed his lifeline and was admiring the view, seemingly unfazed by the height. I inched over and introduced myself.

He told me his name was Maki Koga. He was in his early fifties but easily looked a decade younger, tanned and muscular from a career spent outdoors, tending to the shrine.

"Can you see the people down there, taking pictures of the waterfall?" he asked.

I couldn't actually see the pilgrims and tourists down below, because my view downward was cut off by the edge of the cliff. Koga was standing a big stride ahead of me, toes practically on the brink of the abyss, his white robes fluttering in a breeze thrown up by the mists rising from the basin far below. I forced myself to step a little closer. A baby step, more a shuffle, is all I could manage. I still couldn't see the people. They must have looked like ants from this height.

"Aren't you afraid, Koga-san?" I asked.

"Not at all."

"How do you feel?"

"Grateful," he replied with a big smile.

As we gazed into the blue sky together, I suddenly recalled how frustrated I had been at the bottom of the falls ten years earlier, when I was struggling to comprehend and convey all the spiritual lessons I had absorbed.

"What does Shinto mean to you?" I found myself asking Koga.

"It means being flexible," he answered, without missing a beat. "You know the phrase 'eight million kami'? I love that description. It means there are limitless ways to show your gratitude."

The ceremony that Koga and his fellow priests conducted had been in the Shinto style. But that didn't mean the waters swirling around their feet, or even the falls themselves, were Shinto holy ground—or not Shinto holy ground alone. Nachi Falls is a majestic sight. But it does not manifest out of nowhere. Farther upstream, leading deep into what is known as the Nachi Primeval Forest, can be found another, smaller waterfall, and above it another, and another—some sixty in all, of various sizes. Forty-eight of them have names.

When you go down the list, you see names inspired not only by Shinto but also Shugendo, which in turn incorporate Buddhism and other belief systems from the Asian mainland, Confucian and Taoist, the yin and yang, arcane divinations. For more than a thousand years, seekers of all sorts sought out this rugged terrain, performing rituals and meditating in the chilly mountain waters of what was known as the Forty-Eight Falls beyond Nachi to clear their minds and purify their souls.

In Japan, sacred mountains, Kumano included, have long been known as "shi to saisei no chi"—"a place where one might die and be reborn." Not literally, of course (though those who made the arduous trek to Kumano on foot in the olden days may have felt it more keenly than those of us blessed with modern transport). What the phrase means is that natural habitats give us different perspectives. Even long before modern times, people realized this. Some think of nature as being in opposition to civilization. But in truth they are parts of the same whole. Our civilization exists amid nature, after all, even if it doesn't feel that way inside our air-conditioned homes in our cities and suburbs.

The famous astronomer Carl Sagan once directed a space probe to take an image of Earth from a distance of billions of miles away. Our planet, filled with joy and despair and dramas that seem universe-size to us, resembled a tiny speck from this vantage—"a mote of dust suspended in a sunbeam," as he would later put it. The image is known as the Pale Blue Dot, and its power comes from how it puts us in our place. It reminds us that while we have built great civilizations, we are also clinging to a pebble floating in the infinity of space. It's easy to forget this in the midst of our hectic modern lives, as we strive to function as members of society. Sometimes the negatives are overwhelming, and when this happens, it can feel like the whole world is ending. But the world goes on. That photo of the Pale Blue Dot reminds us that our hopes and fears and furies are actually playing out on what is, comparatively speaking, but a speck of dust in the universe. When you start thinking about life on those scales—and we do live on them, even if we don't directly experience them—it can help ease your load. It might even bring you a smile.

This is what death and rebirth means. It means stripping away what is holding you back, letting you emerge as something new. New perspectives give us new ideas and new values. And this is a process, not a destination. That's why Emperor Go-Shirakawa of old made the journey to Kumano some forty times after abdicating the throne, trying to find himself in the wilds, almost a thousand years ago. That journey's start is waiting for you, whenever you feel lost. And you don't need a space probe to take this path. You don't even need mountains or waterfalls. Just as head priest Kuki told that delegation of visitors to his grand shrine, you can make a connection in whatever little way you can. Like I did when I took that walk in a city park, desperately trying to pull myself together after my mother's death. I experienced my own rebirth, of sorts, as the raven led my eye to the shrine, the trees, the stumps, and the shoots rising up like little fingers from the moss below.

That taught me that I wasn't ever really alone. But it took

a visit to Kumano to remind me that I didn't have to shoe-horn myself into a box, culturally or spiritually or any other way. I can incorporate different aspects of cultures into something new: myself, as I wanted to be. That's the tenderness of which Kuki spoke, I think. And that's the tenderness with which I want to live my life.

CHAPTER 9

Prayer and Play: Asobi

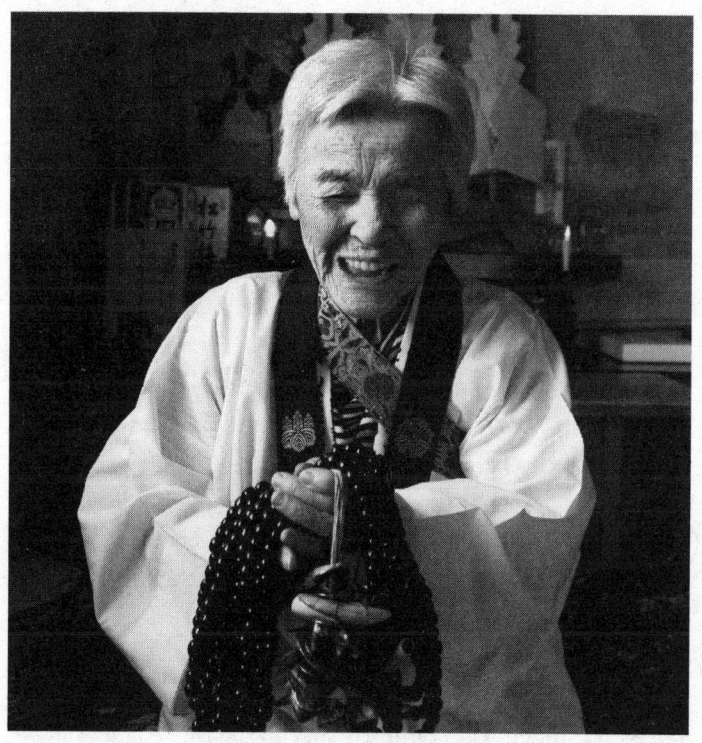

Také Nakamura, the last itako.

Fortune comes in by a merry gate.

—Japanese proverb

We do not have ideology. We do not have theology. We dance.

—Shinto priest quoted in *The Masks of God*

Why is she playing? Why are the eight million kami laughing?

—Amaterasu, Kami of the Sun

month or so after a baby is born in Japan, their parents and grandparents take them to a Shinto shrine to express gratitude for the safe birth and to pray for the child's continued health and happiness. Traditionally, either the mother or grandmother holds the infant, wrapping themselves together in a single kimono (blue for boys, red for girls) to make this first introduction of a new life to the kami. This is called hatsumiya-mairi, literally "one's first visit to a shrine," and is precisely where the "born Shinto" part of the "born Shinto, marry Christian, die Buddhist" mindset comes from.

As it so happens, my parents didn't follow the custom with me. This is a perfect example of the flexibility of Japanese spirituality. They had a choice, and chose for whatever reason not to go. I would be two before I made my first shrine visit, and it is a bit of a funny story.

Traditionally, of course, parents have to carry their newborns to "meet" the kami on that first visit. But I was big enough by that point to toddle on my own two feet. And did I walk! My father always said I walked more than any baby he'd ever seen. I must have really impressed him, as he mentioned it so often over the years. I still love walking today. I almost never take the escalator when stairs are available, or a taxi if the distance is even remotely walkable. When I'm on vacation I inevitably rack up some seriously impressive step counts.

Right around the time I started walking, my parents took me on a trip from our home in Tokyo to Kagawa, on the island of Shikoku. I don't know why they picked this relatively far-flung region for a vacation. But Kagawa is known for its seafood, its udon noodles, and its hot springs, so why not?

At some point, they took me to one of Kagawa's major tourist spots: Kotohira-gu. It's a Shinto shrine with a thousand years of history. It's also known by the nickname Konpira-san, which is taken from the name of the kami once worshipped there, Konpira-Gongen, the Avatar of Konpira. Not so very long ago, this was a Shugendo mountain, said to be filled with tengu, those raven-like familiars of the yamabushi from Japanese folklore. The famed artist Hiroshige captured the scene in one of his *Fifty-Three Stations of the Tokaido,* where a pilgrim in white robes is seen from behind as he approaches the shrine, shouldering a box containing a huge tengu mask, its crimson face staring impassively back the way he came. The faithful approached Konpira in the olden days with a tengu watching their back. I write this in the past tense because the Japanese government ordered the avatar disenshrined in the nineteenth century, with that misguided policy of forcibly stripping anything smacking of Buddhism or Shugendo from Shinto sites. Today Kotohira-gu is ostensibly a Shinto shrine, though tellingly, people still call it Konpira-san to this very day.

The signs of Shugendo may have been stripped away, but you can still touch that history, or more precisely, walk it.

Kotohira-gu sits halfway up Mount Zozu, at the top of an enormous staircase consisting of close to eight hundred stone steps. The natural slope wasn't regraded to fit the steps; the steps were carefully sized to fit nature's curves. As a result the staircase is constructed out of dozens of smaller flights, some shorter, some longer, some steeper, some shallower. From certain vantage points, especially from the top, it almost resembles a ski jump. And then it continues farther up behind Kotohira-gu's main hall, all the way to the mountaintop. There's another shrine there, where visitors can buy a good-luck charm shaped like a tengu's face—the legacy of that long-ago mountain religion. When you stand at the top, looking out over the city far below, with a forest breeze rustling your hair, it's easy to feel like a tengu has your back, just like the pilgrims of yore.

"The moment you saw those stairs, you wanted to walk them," my dad would reminisce. "Your mom and I thought you'd get tired and give up soon enough, but were we wrong!" he'd laugh. "Every time we tried to carry you, you refused!" With my hand in one of theirs, I tromped up the stairs on chubby little legs. Many people passed us, my father said, and the shopkeepers who ran the souvenir shops along the way cheered me on. Everyone was impressed. Eventually, we reached a point where the stairs grew steep enough to start making my parents nervous, and my father carried me up the final stretch by piggyback.

That is the story of my first visit to a Shinto shrine, and I absolutely love it. But interestingly, my parents never framed it in those terms. They didn't see this as a pilgrimage or a ritual. They went to Kotohira-gu because it was famous, and they thought it would be fun. I'm sure they prayed at the top, for my health and our happiness as a family. But Kotohira-gu was merely one sightseeing stop on a longer vacation. This style of traveling is very common in Japan, where prayer and play mix. In fact, it's the default for how we engage with spirituality on an everyday basis. Prayer and play are woven together like threads in a loom here, intertwining the spiritual into the fabric of daily life. Play doesn't mean anything goes—holy grounds are still holy grounds, deserving of basic respect and etiquette. But prayer and play offer another way of interacting with things spiritual: not out of obligation or duty but as a means to refresh yourself.

This helps explain why in Japan, despite it regularly making those least-religious lists, shrines and temples are such tourist draws. They are holy sites, of course. But they are also places to relax and play, in a respectful way.

If you open virtually any travel website, guidebook, or pamphlet about Japan, you'll inevitably see shrines and temples highlighted as places to visit, right alongside natural attractions, restaurants, hotels, and all that. I love touring Japan myself, enjoying great views, savoring local delicacies, spending the night in ryokan inns, soaking in the hot springs, and shopping for fun souvenirs. But it's impossible to imagine going somewhere without visiting temples and shrines. And I'm not alone. A great many people spend their leisure time in Japan this way, residents and visitors both, those of faith and those without. And, in fact, this style of tourism isn't anything new.

The general pattern was already well established centuries ago. Back in the Edo Era, which is the beginning of the seventeenth through the mid-nineteenth century (1603–1868, to be exact), Japanese citizens didn't enjoy the freedom of movement they do today. The shogunate, which ruled all of Japan, strictly controlled all travel. There were checkpoints placed in strategic transport hubs, on major roads, on the borders of cities and territories, and at river and seaports. They functioned something like customs authorities at airports to-day: tracking movement in and out of places, taking taxes, and checking for contraband. There was a famous saying, "Guns coming and women going," meaning the top things agents looked for were guns smuggled in and women trying to get out, which should tell you all you need to know about how women were treated in this era. Travelers needed documents, which listed their address, purpose, and name of whoever issued the permit, kind of like a modern passport. Samurai applied for papers from the feudal government. Average folks applied through whichever Buddhist temple they were regis-tered as a parishioner. (If you'll recall from earlier in the book, registering at a temple was compulsory in those days.)

It wasn't easy to secure permission to travel. But there was one exception: pilgrimage. If your purpose was visiting a shrine or a temple, your papers were almost sure to be ap-proved. One of the most famous of these pilgrim-travelers was a haiku master named Matsuo Basho. In the late seven-teenth century, he applied for papers to take a meandering trip through a series of holy sites deep in the countryside. Travel was dangerous at this time in history; bandits stalked the roads, shaking down travelers for valuables. Basho dressed in monk's robes to make himself a less palatable target for robbers, and also to ease his passing through the many check-points he would encounter. He published his travelogue in 1702 as *The Narrow Road to the Interior*. Virtually every page of his book mentions some temple, shrine, or holy spot.

Basho's much-read classic set the stage for a boom in reli-gious travel. By the early nineteenth century, travel emerged as a major genre in the publishing world, in the form of il-lustrated prints, guidebooks, and fiction set on the road. The most famous of the latter was an 1802 novel titled *To-kaidochu Hizakurige*, or *Tokaido on Two Legs*. It starred a pair of lovable idiots named Yaji and Kita, who lost everything in a get-rich-quick scheme, then applied for papers for a pilgrimage down the Tokaido Road, the foot highway linking the capital of Edo to Kyoto. They planned to visit Ise Grand Shrine in hopes of changing their luck but spent far more time seeking out saké, women, and song than enlightenment. Their adventures seem to have resonated with readers. By 1830, records show more than four million people paid a visit to Ise Grand Shrine.

A famous saying emerged to describe the trend: "Visiting Ise to take a glance at the Grand Shrine." The difficulty of traveling freely meant that people saw the pilgrimage to Ise as a once-in-a-lifetime experience. So they made sure to make the most of their travel papers. They may have gone to Ise first, but then kept going beyond their originally intended destination. They might swing through big cities like Nara, Kyoto, and Osaka, seeing the sights, tasting the local delicacies, meeting the locals. In the sequel to *Tokaido on Two Legs*, Yaji and Kita made it all the way to Konpira-gu, where I went as a toddler. It is more than 250 miles from their supposed destination of Ise.

As Basho wrote in his travelogue, "Every day is a journey, and the journey itself is home." The official purpose for people's peregrinations may have been spiritual, but for many, the sheer pleasure of traveling itself was an equal or greater motivator. This was pilgrimage as recreation.

And the more people traveled, the more they wanted to remember their trips. They wanted souvenirs. Shrines and temples were the first to realize the monetary potential of pilgrimages, and began selling amulets, charms, and talismans to visitors. But some travelers wanted more. Locals began tapping into this demand by selling their own good luck charms to visitors. A great many traditional souvenirs still on sale today have their roots in this pilgrim economy. The colorful wooden figurines known as kokeshi dolls are one such example. Different regions developed their own products. Aizu artisans created toys called Akabeko, a wooden figurine shaped like an ox, covered in bright red papier-mâché. The town of Otsu, just outside of Kyoto, did a brisk business in Otsu-é, literally "Otsu pictures," folk paintings sold as talismans for various needs, ranging from preventing fire to ensuring abundant harvests. Painted with bold brushstrokes, they're almost cartoonlike, such as a variety featuring monstrous oni, or ogres, dressed in monks' robes.

When the American businessman Francis Hall first came to Japan in 1859, only a few years had passed since the nation's ports opened to the outside world. He noted in his journal just how lively Japan's holy spots were. Of a temple in Kanagawa, just southwest of Tokyo, he wrote that "on either side of the principal temple gate were rows of refreshment tables, stands of confectionery, fancy articles of dress such as hairpins, tobacco pouches, combs, and children's toys innumerable. Each table was besieged by a crowd of little traffickers."

The crowds of "traffickers," little and big, never really stopped their "sieges." This is why the roads leading to shrines and temples today are often packed with shops selling snacks and souvenirs, tea and toys. The Nakamise shopping arcade, which leads to Sensoji Temple in Tokyo, is a textbook example. It is one of the oldest purveyors of these spiritual souvenirs, dating back to the seventeenth century.

I can't even count how many times I've visited Sensoji over the years, but I never get tired of it, because of this dynamic mix of prayer and play. The fun begins the moment you pass through the entrance of Kaminarimon, the enormous crimson "Thunder Gate." Beyond it lies a shopping arcade some 820 feet long, both sides packed with little shops, with virtu-

ally no space between. This is the Nakamise, and it sells all
sorts of things. Many are purported to bring good luck to
those who purchase them. Beckoning cats—those feline figurines with a paw raised to rake in fortune—are everywhere,
of course. But my favorites are the foods.

If you have a sweet tooth, as I do, this stretch of Tokyo is
a little slice of heaven on earth. Asakusa's trademark dessert
is a sweet concoction of crispy puffed rice and sugar, kind
of like a hard Rice Krispie Treat. They're called kaminari
okoshi, literally "thunder-crackers," a callback to the entrance gate, and, according to those who sell them, an auspicious thing to eat when launching a new endeavor of some
kind. Sponge cakes called ningyo-yaki, which means "baked
dolls," are another Asakusa specialty. These little pastries
are molded in all sorts of shapes: a turtle symbolizing longevity, a five-storied pagoda, or the smiling faces of the
Seven Gods of Happiness, to name a few. Some are filled
with custard, others with anko, a sweet paste made from
azuki beans, themselves an auspicious food because their
crimson color is said to drive evil spirits away.

But my favorite of all is zenzai, a sweet red bean soup
served with mochi rice cakes or dango dumplings, their
delicately nutty rice flavor and chewiness contrasting beautifully with the rich sweetness of the broth. There are competing theories as to how it got its name. One is that *zenzai*
is a Buddhist term of praise. The other is that *zenzai* sounds
like *jinzai*, a reading of the kanji for "kami are here," which
evokes the name of a festival in Izumo when all eight million kami of Japan are said to be in attendance at Izumo
Grand Shrine. The hodgepodge of Japan's spirituality, in the
form of a dessert.

Of a visit to Asakusa in the spring of 1860, Hall wrote:
"Thither flock pilgrims from all parts of the empire to make

their offerings and pay their vows . . . From the first to the second gateway, a distance of several hundred feet, the walk was one impacted mass of people . . . And on either side of the walk were continuous rows of booths, for the sale of small wares such as the distant pilgrim might purchase as mementoes of his visit." Hall was particularly impressed by the toys, which he said "occupied by far the greater part of the space."

There's an old saying that goes, "Children are in the hands of the kami until they turn seven." Way back when, lifespans were much shorter due to the low standard of medical care. Up to 30 percent of children perished at a very young age from illness or disease, making the age of seven a very real milestone. Parents doted on their youngsters, treating them to presents as they took them to temples and shrines to pray for their continued health. The song "Toryanse" ("You May Pass"), which you can hear playing at many a crosswalk in Japan today, is actually another example of spirituality in plain sight. The song is a few hundred years old. The lyrics are about passing through a checkpoint—a pilgrimage, by parents visiting a shrine to thank the kami for their child's seventh birthday:

> *You may pass. You may pass.*
> *Where does this narrow path lead?*
> *This path goes to Tenjin shrine.*
> *Please let us pass, let us pass.*
> *Only those with good reason may pass.*
> *We're returning a talisman to celebrate this*
>   *child turning seven.*
> *Going is easy. Returning is scary.*
> *You may be scared, but you may pass.*

Many traditional toys have a spiritual component, serving double duty as good-luck charms. The spinning of tops is said to drive evil spirits away; the flying of kites, a prayer for children to soar. There's an old game called fuku-warai (lucky laughter), in which you wear a blindfold and try to stick facial features onto a blank face. It's kind of like pin the tail on the donkey, but the point isn't to make the perfect face. It's to make the funniest one. And it's played with the faces of kami: Otafuku, a chubby-cheeked goddess of fortune, and Hyottoko, said to protect homes against fire. Francis Hall would have seen all these on his visit, and while he was right that they were for children, it was more likely that families played with them together.

"Fortune comes in by a merry gate" goes another Japanese proverb. And that's spirituality here in a nutshell. People visit shrines and temples for edification and guidance, for support and solace, but also simply for pleasure, the expression of fun becoming a sort of sacrament in and of itself. I was too little to remember my first family trip to Kotohira-gu shrine, but I'm sure about one thing: We all had a good time.

To approach spirituality with a playful mindset is to cultivate joy. In our spiritual traditions, we play because it's fun to sing or dance, or even shop on one of those arcades leading to a holy spot, but also because it's important: It helps to refresh and reset, to nourish a positive mindset. That goes beyond worship or faith. It is a perspective. One that helps us live.

The word for play in Japanese is *asobi*. It's the word we use for having fun with toys, with children, with friends. But it wasn't always used this way. Long ago, *asobi* meant something spiritual: interacting with the kami. Specifically, it meant to dance.

EVERYBODY LOVES A GOOD PARTY. THE KAMI ARE NO EX-
ception. You can make a convincing argument that they
taught the world to party.

Japan's first and most famous party is portrayed in the
Kojiki. In a fit of pique, Amaterasu, the kami of the sun, hid
herself away in a cave, and the rest of the eight million kami
gathered to lure her out of seclusion. They conducted rituals, enlisted the help of sacred animals, recited liturgies.
But in the end, it was a dance that saved the day, a dance so
entertaining that it caused the assembled kami to erupt in
raucous laughter. A solemn ritual didn't get Amaterasu to
poke her head out and light up the world again. It was a
dance.

To this day, dance is treated as a sacrament in Shinto. In
spite of its mythical origins in that wild dance party of the
kami, it isn't a free-form thing; it is always performed as
part of a solemn ceremony. It's called kagura, and is written
with the characters that mean "pleasing the kami." The musical rhythms and footwork are ancient, requiring long
study to perfect. There are many forms, many regional
variations. But the most common is known as miko-mai, or
"shrine maiden's dance." To perform it one must be a miko:
a shrine maiden.

In English, "shrine maiden" sounds like something out of
fantasy or folklore, but in practice it is very down-to-earth
work. And it is work: Shrines pay a salary, and it isn't uncommon for them to take out want ads for the position. A
miko's routine involves assisting the shrine's priest in their
daily rituals, working at the shop that sells talismans and
charms to visitors, and sweeping up around the grounds.
(You may have heard of this last part through cleaning guru
Marie Kondo, who cites having worked as a miko as part of

her origin story.) Miko also serve as dancers in special ceremonies, where kagura dances are offered up to entertain
the kami. Not every miko studies shrine dance—it's a special skill. But to perform a shrine dance, you generally need
to be a miko.

I'd always been curious about miko. They are hard to
miss. They dress in distinctive white and crimson attire,
tying back their locks of jet-black hair with intricate arrangements of paper and ribbon. The undyed hair and the
lack of makeup and piercings, all modern affectations forbidden for miko on duty, make them seem like something
out of another era, which in a sense they are.

Priests typically inherit their positions, which are passed
down along the bloodlines of the families that run the shrines.
But miko tend to be hired from among young women who
live in the surrounding community. My impression was that
miko tended to be in their late teens or early twenties. As an
adult, it never even occurred to me to apply for the job.

But then something funny happened. I'd become interested in gagaku, the ancient court music that is the accompaniment to kagura dancing. Typically, it is performed using
an ensemble of instruments: biwa (lutes), sho (mouth or-
gans), hichiriki (oboes), ryuteki (dragon flutes), and a variety of traditional drums. I decided to study the dragon flute,
and spent many hours taking lessons and practicing at
home. At some point during one of my classes, the topic of
miko shrine maidens came up. My instructor mentioned
that there is no official age limit. When I expressed surprise, she offered to introduce me to a master of miko-mai
shrine dance. This sensei was seventy-nine years old, my
instructor said, and had learned the dances as a teenager,
when she herself had been a miko. Now shrines sent their
miko to her, to learn the rhythms and footwork.

So it was that I found myself commuting to her classroom once a week. It was held in a large practice space on the grounds of a shrine in the suburbs of western Tokyo. This being a shrine dance studio, it was decorated in the Japanese style, sliding fusuma panels for walls and shoji paper screens for windows, surrounding a large open space covered in tatami mats. They filled the room with a faint, clean fragrance of grass. The elderly sensei was soft-spoken and petite. She moved slowly, but her posture was perfectly straight, the benefit of a lifetime spent dancing, I supposed. She taught a small group of students, five or maybe six at most. I was the only one not sent to her by a shrine.

While happy at the prospect of a new student, she was surprised to learn that I was there of my own volition. But I was determined. For months I studied—or more accurately, mimicked. There weren't really any "lessons." Sensei would put on a recording of a gagaku song and dance while I attempted to follow her movements, or I would stand behind a more experienced dancer and imitate them. There didn't seem to be any "steps," in the way of a waltz or tango or what have you. The performance was a series of turns and glides, tabi-stockinged feet sliding over tatami worn smooth by countless students before me, punctuated by precisely timed jingles of a kagura-suzu, a conical "tree" of handbells. From the bells' grip trailed long, colorful ribbons that one had to take great care not to become tangled up in as one danced. When I made a mistake, which was often, sensei would glide in and correct me by physically adjusting my arm or foot. The movements were slow, deliberate, and controlled. Always controlled. You couldn't overthink it, though, or even really think at all. The minute you tried to inject yourself into the mix, you'd mess up. It was less expressing yourself than it was expressing patterns, or even instincts. "This isn't about making an impression," sensei would say. "Move like a hawk circles in the sky."

A little under a year after I began, I had a surprise. Sensei asked me to perform at the shrine that hosted her classroom. The occasion was the reitaisai, an annual ceremony to thank the kami. It would involve kagura, and they needed a solo dancer. I wasn't a miko, but sensei's recommendation was credential enough, it seemed. I'd been studying shrine dance out of curiosity, and while the idea I might participate in a shrine ceremony had entered my mind, I'd assumed I'd be part of a larger group. The thought of performing all on my own struck terror into my heart. I agreed, but I barely slept for a week after. Over and over, I imagined making a mistake onstage.

The ceremony was held at the end of August, a sweltering season in Tokyo. My performance was "Urayasu-no-mai"—"The Dance of Tranquility." It is the most well known kagura; if you see miko performing at a Shinto shrine, chances are it is this dance. It is about ten minutes long and consists of two parts. The first half involves a traditional hi-ogi, a fancy folding fan with blades made of fragrant hinoki cypress, with long colorful threads trailing from either side. The second half utilizes that kagura-suzu, the bells I mentioned. They look something like a ceremonial mace, with fifteen small bells about the size of grapes arranged in tiers on the top, and long multicolored ribbons extending from the bottom of the grip. Shaken with precise flicks of the wrist, it produces a distinctive jangle that is believed to drive negative energies away—a sort of sonic purifier.

I threw myself into practicing, almost frantically so. I

wasn't sleeping or eating well. Eventually, I reached a sort of breaking point. I pulled aside the most experienced student to confess my fears—and, potentially, even ask to find a replacement. I told her how inadequate I felt, that I knew any one of my fellow students would make a better choice than me. I didn't want to embarrass myself or anyone else. But her reply stopped me short.

"You keep saying you're worried about people. About yourself, about sensei and the other students, about those who come to watch on the day of the performance. But you have the wrong idea. You aren't doing this for us. You're doing this for the kami."

She explained, "It's true the others dance better than you. They have years of experience to your months. But sensei isn't looking for the ultimate dancer. She saw you, and how hard you've been practicing. And she thought that spirit better suited this year's ceremony. It isn't about who's most skilled. It's about heart. And that's why she wants you to offer your kagura dance to the kami."

This was precisely what I needed to hear. It was true: shrine dancing was a performance, but it wasn't like a dance recital. It wasn't for the pleasure of the assembled, not the priest or the parishioners or even the dancer themselves. It was for the kami. That was the only audience I needed to think about.

On the day of the performance, sensei and the other students helped me into my costume, a version of the robes worn by ladies-in-waiting in the Japanese imperial court more than a thousand years ago. This was the very first time I'd ever worn anything like it. Kagura costumes are expensive; this was my teacher's, too elaborate and precious to use in practice sessions. Layers of fabric constricted my chest; a long train, like that of a Western wedding dress, added unfamiliar weight to my waist.

This particular shrine venerated Susano'o, Amaterasu's wild younger brother. You might remember him from the very first chapter: He's the one who so infuriated the sun goddess that she plunged the world into permanent darkness. It might seem odd to venerate a troublemaker, but in fact that is the entire point. Susano'o isn't a "bad guy," to distill it to a childish term. He is the prototypical aratama, a wild spirit, powerful and mercurial. He may have sown great mischief in the high plains of the heavens, but after being banished to the mortal realm, he used his great powers to free us from the Orochi, a monster that *Chronicles of Japan* describes in vivid terms:

> It had an eight-forked head and an eight-forked tail;
>   its eyes were red, like the winter-cherry;
>   and on its back evergreens were growing.
>   In its undulations its body filled eight hills and
> eight valleys.

The Orochi is a monster, but its description evokes the sensation of a natural disaster. To me it sounds like a mudslide. In the *Chronicles* it menaces humanity, consuming our children until Susano'o slays it. It's a thrilling story with a quiet message: The things that terrify us can also liberate us. It's all a matter of context. Susano'o is the proverbial double-edged sword.

So I put the parishioners out of my mind. I put the shrine priest out of my mind. I even put sensei out of my mind. This, what I was about to do, was entirely for Susano'o, enfant terrible of the high plains of the heavens.

I'd practiced hard, for many weeks, in the studio. And I'd continued after coming home. I'd had my husband remove a ceiling light in our bedroom, the only room in the house with tatami floors, to give me more room to raise my arms. I'd wrapped a bedsheet around my waist to simulate the train I'd have to avoid tripping over as I twirled. I'd honestly done everything I could do to prepare, and now there was nothing to do other than dance. Whatever else might happen was up to the kami.

On the big day, I wouldn't be dancing in a classroom or a stage; I would be performing in front of the altar of the shrine. As parishioners filed in and took seats on folding stools inside, I waited on the veranda for my cue to enter and begin my performance. The scheduled time arrived and went. A classmate darted in and out of the shrine, giving me updates that consisted of little more than "not quite yet." A half hour passed, then an hour. What happened? There was nothing to do but let it go. I was in that mindset I call kami territory—both metaphorically, in that I knew whatever was delaying things was out of my hands, and literally, in that I was standing on the grounds of a Shinto shrine. This helped me remain calm, even as temperatures rose both figuratively and literally.

Later, I would learn that an elderly audience member had fainted from low blood sugar, and the delay was due to their calling an ambulance to take him to the hospital. But I didn't know any of this at the time. I suspect my "assistant" didn't tell me because she knew it didn't matter—there was nothing to do but wait. And then, finally, came the cue.

I honestly don't remember much about my performance other than it went off without a hitch. I don't know if my dance was as smooth as "a hawk circles in the sky," but I like to think that it went well enough to please the audience it was intended for: Susano'o. Later, my teacher told me she'd heard from the head priest that I did a good job, and that was that.

I've since "retired" from shrine dancing, for a variety of reasons. Dance is a very physical art form, but when I look back, it is the mental aspects of training and performing that most stay with me. When I agreed to perform publicly, I honestly thought I was out of my league, that I was biting off more than I could chew. And truly, I was making an honest assessment of what I thought my capabilities were. But in hindsight, I now know that this kind of thinking was only holding me back. My burning desire to do my best was a powerful motivator. But it also fueled a monster within me. I know this sounds melodramatic. It may not have had eight heads and eight tails, like the one Susano'o faced, but it possessed the very real capability to send shivers of fear down my spine, every bit as visceral as if I'd been cornered by some sort of beast in real life.

Shrine dancing made me realize that the person driving myself into that corner wasn't really a monster, but me. Our own hopes and desires fuel our fears and anxieties. Like Susano'o, all of us are double-edged swords. The only one telling me *you aren't good enough* was me. Such a simple phrase, yet with such power to thwart and bind, almost like a magical spell. It made me start wondering how many times I'd sabotaged myself with it, how many opportunities I'd missed. There's a famous quote that sometimes doing your best isn't good enough. But my dance at the shrine taught me that isn't right at all. Doing your best *is* good enough—and whatever happens beyond that is in kami territory. Once you've done your best to prepare, there's no good or bad, pass or fail.

There's just doing—meaning that whatever happens will be a new experience, and experiences, both positive and negative, are the real currency of our lives.

....

MOST WILL NEVER GET TO EXPERIENCE "PLAYING" WITH THE kami through traditional dance, as ritualized and formal as it is. But there is another sort of dance in which anyone can participate, one that is both spiritual and downright fun. It is called bon-odori, the bon dance. We do it every summer. The specific dates and scale of these Obon festivals, as they're known, vary from place to place, but this is a tradition with a long history—the Japanese have been celebrating it in various forms for five centuries now.

Obon fuses two strands of spiritual thought: an indigenous belief in ancestral kami and an imported Buddhist custom of honoring the spirits of one's ancestors. It is a time when the borders between the worlds of living and dead blur, when the spirits return to their old homes in the world of the living for a brief time. We place small bonfires outside the entrances of our homes, beacons for the dearly departed to find their way back. We construct figurines, sticking toothpicks into cucumbers and eggplants, to create shapes symbolizing horses and oxen, the former so that the spirits might save time by racing home quickly, the latter so that they might return to the land of the dead more slowly. But most of all, we dance.

When I was growing up, bon-odori was always one of the highlights of my summer. As a child I never put much thought into the spiritual aspects, to be honest. There was still a big, empty dirt lot in our neighborhood, and that's where the community association held the festival every July. The preparation would begin the day before, as local men erected a temporary scaffold in the middle of the lot, two stories tall, its topmost platform big enough to hold a large wadaiko drum, upon which our neighbors would take turns beating out the rhythms of the festivities to come. From the platform's corners they strung streamers and lines of paper lanterns, each lit from within by a light bulb to illuminate the name of a resident or local business who'd contributed to sponsor the event. Wooden stalls would appear on the edges of the space, where local mom-and-pop storekeepers would sell all sorts of fun stuff: cotton candy, kakigori (shaved ice), and glimmering anzu-ame (apricots enrobed in translucent candy-syrup), colorful water balloons you'd bounce on a rubber band like yo-yos, and plastic masks of cartoon characters. There were all sorts of carnival games, like kingyo-sukui, where you'd try to scoop up shimmering goldfish from kiddie pools before your paper net dissolved in the water. I'd get excited just watching the preparations unfold.

The festival would start at 6:00 p.m., but nobody watched the clock. I'd listen for the music and wait for the drums, each strike resonating over the rooftops, the cue to tug on my mother's sleeve to take my sister and me over, for my father would inevitably still be at work. Along the way we'd join with neighbors, the kids positively bouncing as we made our way to the festival lot. The parents wore their usual clothes, but they put us in traditional yukata robes and geta sandals, making us little time travelers from a bygone era, clad in soft cotton and shod in smooth wood. We weren't used to this footwear, which felt like flip-flops made of stiff boards and were hard to walk in, but I loved the satisfying clops they made on the concrete: *Karan-koron! Karan-koron!* When I was little, the sound of geta signaled fun to come. I still love wearing them today, whenever I get the chance.

There were many ways to enjoy a bon-odori. But dancing

was my favorite. There's music specifically written for festival dancing, classics as familiar to us as Christmas carols are to Americans, with a lot more regional variations. The organizers would pick a series of songs for the evening, ranging from old classics to newer versions based on popular anime theme songs, to appeal to participants of every age group. They'd play recordings over loudspeakers, with the drummer providing a supplementary background beat on the wadaiko. The languid rhythms were a perfect fit for a sultry summer evening, slow and repetitive and inviting, all the better for anyone to join in the dance. Middle-aged women dressed in matching yukata, like uniforms, would lead the dances, assembling in a circle around the central tower to encourage the rest of us to join in. They'd been practicing and knew the traditional dances well. The footwork was designed for those wearing yukata, which keep the legs close together, so there were no high-steps, just leisurely sashays around the circle, feet sweeping and arms waving to the drumbeat. The rest of us would slide into the ring at an opportune moment and mimic their practiced moves from behind, laughing at our flailing discombobulation as we tried to keep up. The emcees would usually play a tune twice in succession, partly so amateurs could get in a "practice round," partly to simply enjoy a fun song again.

My favorite was titled "The 21st Century Dance." It told the story of a young couple wondering if they would still be together in what was, when the song first came out in 1969, the far future: three decades ahead, at the dawn of the twenty-first century. It was bright and poppy, with footwork just a little faster than in classic bon-odori songs. Whenever I heard the first bars come over the speakers, I'd jump up and shout. I'd hand my sticky cotton candy to my mother and rush into the circle. These neighborhood dances are like a form of interactive performance art, to be joined in rather than watched. The participation is the point: Nobody is at the center of attention; and there's no expectation that anyone really be good—just have a good time. The lyrics of the "Awa Odori," which is sung in the Tokushima region, capture the spirit really well. Their titular song goes "It's a fool who dances and a fool who watches; if both are fools, you might as well dance."

The bon-odori is, for all intents and purposes, a secular festival today, a chance for neighbors to gather and celebrate a midsummer's eve together. But it originated in a form of play that was a literal matter of life and death. Our ancient ancestors believed that for the souls of the departed to reach the hereafter, they needed to be entertained. *Chronicles of Japan* contains a scene where a young kami dies, and his wife and parents build a "mourning hut" where they played—not prayed, but played, in that very old sense of the word. For eight days and nights, they drank and sang and danced to musical accompaniment. The custom seems to have been well established by the third century, for there's a manuscript written by a Chinese visitor from the era describing such scenes. The history of bon-odori is long and braided; this might be called the Shinto strand of its "cultural DNA."

There's another strand, more recent, that can be traced back to a Buddhist monk named Ippen, who lived in the 1200s. He was a wandering holy man who eschewed organized religion. He sought a simpler path, the better to lead the average man and woman to salvation. His method was teaching them to chant the sutra "namu-amida-butsu," which translates into something like "I trust in the merciful Buddha." Now, this in and of itself wasn't particularly unique; it was the doctrine of the Pure Land sect of Buddhism, and the phrase is well known and used in Japan even today. But Ippen developed a distinctive style of reciting it, dancing as he sang it aloud. This kind of performance was all but unheard of among the Buddhist clergy, and the sight of a monk twirling and dancing as he sang the sutras began to draw delighted crowds. As his fame grew, so did his retinue of followers, who traveled with him, singing and dancing and converting more locals. They would erect stages when they arrived in a place, situating Ippen in the middle, forming a circle, and then dancing around him—sound familiar?

Ippen died in 1289. The records say he danced right up until the very end. His passing ended his performances. But it seems they left quite an impression, for many of the places he visited so enjoyed the singing and dancing that they decided to keep it up for themselves. Over the years it evolved from ritual into a sort of entertainment—but not just any entertainment. In the era of the traditional lunisolar calendar, people all over Japan would stay up all night every July 15 and dance under the light of the full moon, because they believed that their ancestors would drop by for a visit, riding in on the moonbeams. Life was hard then, and this was one of the few occasions when ordinary folks might gather for a bit of unbridled fun.

Some of these parties evolved into pageants, participants one-upping one another with silly costumes. Men might dress as women. Women as men. Some dressed like beggars or nobles. Anything that might grab attention and make the others laugh was fair game. In the nineteenth century, the artist Hiroshige produced a woodblock print of his impression of a long-ago bon-odori. One woman swishes a bamboo branch wildly in the air. Another dancer wears a bucket like a hat. Another dances with a half-eaten watermelon rind tied to his head. All the while an old man beats the drums, setting the rhythm for the fun. These folks really seem to have taken the saying about fools and dancing to heart.

That sort of thing was already old history by the time Hiroshige drew up his illustration. And today, the religious aspects of the event have been mostly lost. But the dance remains, as does the festive atmosphere, a timeless form of play echoing through the centuries. In modern times, bon dances are more like summer block parties.

This is why I don't think of Obon as Buddhist, which isn't to say that it isn't, but neither is it precisely right. I think the better term might be that it's *Japanese* Buddhist. The religion of Buddhism originated in India and came to Japan by way of Korea and China. As it percolated from elite early adopters down through the rungs of society, it evolved and transformed to serve the needs of everyday people. Eventually, it came to center around the deeply rooted native belief of kuyo. Traditional thinking held that the souls of the recently dead were "rough," still connected in some way to the earth, wandering and confused, even potentially harmful to the living. The only way to appease a rough soul so that it might rest in peace was to play with it. So entertained, a rough soul might transform into an ancestor kami, not a deity on high but a kind of guardian angel for a family.

Twenty years and more have passed beyond the millennium that my favorite song was written to commemorate. The old sandlot where the festivals were held is long gone. A construction crew broke ground for an apartment complex there when I was in sixth grade, and I still remember how sad I felt. The old folks who taught us the dances by example, passing down to us the traditions they had learned as children, are gone as well. And so, of course, is my mother, and now my father with her. The bon-odori I danced with a smile, untouched by regret or sadness, exists only in the gauzy haze of fond memory. The neighborhood still dances every year, but the location and faces have changed, with new generations staffing the booths and singing the songs. I'm happy the summer festival continues, even if I miss those old days when I could do it with family and friends.

....

OBON OFFERS US A SYMBOLIC FORM OF COMMUNICATION with the dead. But there is a traditional way to communicate with the dead in more literal terms. Spirit mediums known as itako can be found in the Tohoku region, the far northern reaches of the main island of Japan. Itako aren't ordained, or part of any organized religion; they operate independently, harnessing a mix of spiritual traditions to bridge the here and now and the hereafter, performing a variety of spiritual rituals for the communities they serve. But most of all, they are known for their supposed ability to channel the spirits of the dead.

Traditionally, itako were chosen from the ranks of young women who were either born blind or had lost their sight. Boys would be sent to guilds of the blind, who would train them in "touch-oriented" careers such as massage or acupuncture. Girls who lost their eyesight were sent to the itako. Today, fortunately, it is exceedingly rare for a child to lose their sight to disease, and the numbers of itako are dwindling. As recently as the 1970s, there were around a hundred blind women plying the trade in Aomori. Today, there is only one. There are others who call themselves itako, but she is the only one who is blind and learned the practice according to the old customs. Her name is Také Nakamura. She was ninety years old when I met her. She has no disciples. When she passes, this culture, at least in its traditional form, will pass with her.

There is little written about itako in the English language because they don't neatly slot into any mainstream religious tradition, making them difficult to explain to outsiders. But if you've made it this far, you're in a rare position to understand. So far, you've read of Shinto and Buddhism and Shugendo, of uranai and kuyo, of funerals and ghosts. The itako traffic in all of these things and more, and as you'll see, they do it through a combination of prayer and play. In many ways, they are human manifestations of the hodgepodge of Japanese spirituality.

I'm not the sort of person who consults palm readers or mediums or thinks much about the afterlife in any concrete way. But the itako have always fascinated me, their esoteric spiritual traditions existing just tantalizingly beyond the periphery of the mainstream, at least the mainstream of the places where I was raised and spent my life. Honestly, these mysterious, witchy women are as exotic to a modern urbanite like me as they are to a non-Japanese. I wanted to visit an itako out of curiosity. I chose Nakamura because she was, in many ways, the last of her kind. I hoped to experience a quaint tradition. I thought, perhaps, I might ask her to connect me to my father, just to see how the traditions worked. But things played out quite differently than I'd planned.

I boarded a bullet train from Tokyo on a very chilly morning in December of 2022. At my destination in Aomori, four hours north, waited a local historian who specialized in itako traditions and had edited several books on the topic. He was late-middle-aged, balding, and dressed in khakis and a down jacket. There was nothing about his outward appearance to suggest his unusual interests. I'd found him online and struck up a correspondence. Eventually, he offered to introduce me to Také Nakamura.

We hailed a taxi outside the station. My guide told the

driver we were going to so-and-so village. The driver nodded briskly in recognition.

"I get a lot of requests for that place," he said. "What is it?"

I told him that we were meeting an itako. Again he nodded, wholly unsurprised. Out of curiosity, I asked him if he had ever consulted one himself.

"No," he replied, "but my aunt has, many times." As though it were the most common thing in the world. Which it seemed to be here.

The ride took about an hour. Along the way, the historian delivered a mini lecture on itako. He had strong feelings on the subject and told me there are a lot of itako out there who are itako in name only. There are two criteria for defining a traditional, authentic itako, he continued.

The first is a clear lineage, from a recognized master to the apprentice. Nakamura can trace hers back seven generations, some 250 years.

The second is possessing a rosary of prayer beads and a special talisman called an odaiji, both inherited from their master. Buddhist prayer rosaries are commonplace items in Japan, but they generally range from about six inches to a foot when stretched out. An itako's rosary is unusually long, perhaps six and a half feet, with beads made of dried soapberries that wear smooth after decades of use. At intervals along the strand are additional decorations: boar tusks, fragments of deer horn, and bear claws, all protection against evil, and antique coins, the kind with holes in the center. These symbolize the fare one must pay the ferryman at the River Sanzu, Japan's equivalent of the River Styx, separating our lives from the afterlife. The odaiji is a bamboo tube covered in beautiful silk cloth that is slung across her back, bandolier-style. It contains a fragment of a Buddhist sutra, personally chosen for her by her master. This is said to protect the itako from becoming possessed by malevolent entities or the spirits she channels. An odaiji is a symbol of a professional, full-fledged itako. She always wears her odaiji when doing her job.

Outside the taxi's windows, suburban scenery gave way to rural. Apple groves, Aomori's pride, dormant in winter. A shuttered elementary school, another casualty of Japan's declining birth rate.

"The training takes three to five years," continued the historian. "Apprentices need to memorize around a hundred different sutras, prayers, spells, and rituals. There are a lot of sutras for contacting the kami or Buddhas for health problems: headaches, backaches, toothaches, high blood pressure, any health problems people might have—and also the health of oxen and horses. Livestock were critical for survival here."

He reminds me that their masters were all blind, too. The blind leading the blind, literally. It's difficult for people like us, who spent our whole lives relying on our sight, to imagine how difficult this must have been. There were no written texts. An itako learned everything she knew from careful listening and memorization. And not all of the training was indoors. Some of it was quite extreme: hiking into the mountains to purify oneself under freezing alpine waterfalls, fasting, and such. Neither master nor apprentice could see, which made these difficult tasks even more treacherous. Avoiding injury required them to utilize every sense available to them. This was scary, perilous, even traumatic stuff. From my own research, I'd gathered that some itako chose not to take apprentices because their own training had been so harsh that they couldn't bear to put another young woman through the same.

The historian told me that, centuries back, it was common for itako to marry yamabushi, practitioners of Shugendo. The earliest itako are said to have learned chanting by ear from their husbands, then developed their own styles and methods, which were passed down, again by ear, to their disciples. Which raised a question in my mind.

"How did the itako survive the Meiji Era, when the government was banning Buddhist influences?"

"Because they were seen as miko, shamanesses serving the kami. Také-san, for instance, worships Amaterasu, the Shinto sun goddess."

The taxi pulled into a residential area, then stopped in front of an ordinary private home, absolutely nothing to indicate that a blind shamaness lived within. The historian slid open the front door and called out a greeting.

Soon an elderly woman appeared in the entrance, dressed in a blue-and-white-striped shirt and trousers with a flower pattern. She bowed deeply in welcome. This was Také Nakamura, the last itako. She looked so much like a friendly grandma that I suddenly felt as though I was visiting one of my relatives. So much so that I can't bear to call her by her last name, as journalistic style usually has it. She was most definitely a Také-san.

"Come in, come in," called Také-san. "Warm yourselves up at the kotatsu." Slowly but steadily, she led us into her living room. The three of us took seats around the low heated table, putting our legs and feet under the warmth of its duvet.

"There are tea sets right over there," she said, gesturing in the general direction. "Please make yourselves some tea. I wish I could make it for you, but I'm too old, and I can't see anything at all." Until she said this, I'd forgotten she was blind. It was easy to forget. She moved so smoothly, and when I spoke, she looked directly at my face. When the historian said something, she moved to face him, too. Later, when I took photos of her, she always managed to face my camera, even without my directing her. It seemed her senses were more acute than those of us who could see.

But the more time I spent, the more subtle differences I noticed. Her home was unusually tidy, with nothing on the floor one might trip over. There was no decoration, no ornaments or figurines. This might have simply passed for minimalist decor, but then there was the bathroom, which had no mirror over the sink.

Yet neither did the room feel barren. Her curtains, which kept the chill outside the windows at bay, had pretty flower patterns; the tea set featured a cheerful gingham pattern. Some of the cushions had cute characters on them, picked, I suspected, by her grandchildren. It was the space of someone with family, someone loved and cared for.

I fixed tea for the three of us and took my seat under the kotatsu. Instinctively, I took her hand, telling her what an honor it was to meet her. This was in the midst of the pandemic, and we were supposed to distance, but I didn't know what else to do. Japan is not a handshake culture. Physical touch between strangers is all but unknown. We show appreciation by bowing, and involvement in a conversation by nodding. But she couldn't see any of that. So I took her hand, cool and firm and deeply wrinkled. The touch reminded me of my parents. They would have been around her same age, were they still alive. Memories of walking hand in hand with them, as I had on that long-ago trip to Konpira-gu.

When we finished our tea, she led us into her prayer room. It was small, perhaps thirteen feet on a side. A Shinto-style shimenawa rope festooned with shide paper streamers hung from the ceiling, the dividing line between where we would sit and the sacred place where she would work, a low desk-like table in front of an altar.

The altar was nothing like any home kamidana or butsu-dan, nor did it resemble anything I'd seen in a shrine or temple. On the wall behind the altar hung three vertical scrolls. The middle featured the names of three kami written in bold ink calligraphy, Amaterasu's largest of all. To the right hung a painting of her, to the left a painting of Ta-kasago, a famous pair of kami taking the form of an old couple, representing longevity. Beneath them was a shelf with three elaborately folded paper yorishiro, which serve as temporary receptacles for the kami during rituals. Next to them was a wooden ofuda talisman from Izumo Grand Shrine, where the eight million kami are said to gather for their conclave once every year.

This was Shinto in nature, but in front of this altar stood another table, made of dark wood. Atop it sat a bowl for offerings brought by customers for their loved ones, flanked by electric candles. And just to one side were a pair of hand-made figurines of jizo bodhisattva, those little childlike guardians that are said to watch over travelers everywhere.

At the very bottom sat a low, light-colored wooden desk, the kind one might use in a tatami room, kneeling. Upon it sat a large, black, Buddhist bell, with another pair of candles, these real. This was Také-san's prayer area.

The arrangement was subtle—I could imagine causal observers mistaking it for either Buddhist or Shinto. You'd have to realize Shinto doesn't use candles, for instance, or that Buddhists generally don't put images of Amaterasu in their altars. The mixing of religious symbols had the effect of making the altar seem an empty canvas, allowing those who visited to fill in the blanks with whatever they liked, whatever their beliefs might be. An invitation to the Shinto and Buddhist pantheons both.

Také-san opened a drawer and took out a folded white robe, which she unfurled and put on in one practiced movement. Then she took out her rosary. It was of an impressive length; I'd estimate longer than six feet. At either end of its circumference was a thick "knot" of charms and talismans. I could make out old coins, what appeared to be bear claws, and the lower jawbones of some kind of mammal: a boar, and a deer, perhaps? Or maybe even that of the Japanese wolf, long extinct? Wrapping a chain of beads around one hand, she turned back to face us.

"I'm ready," she said, her sightless eyes somehow finding my own. The grandma with whom I'd just had tea was gone. Before me sat an itako.

"Who would you like me to contact?"

I'd put a lot of thought into whom I might reach out to. Would I ask the medium to connect me with one of the grandparents I'd never met as a little girl? Or perhaps my maternal great-grandfather, the mountain-climbing scientist whose diaries I'd inherited? Or my parents?

My mother was risky business. We quarreled a lot, she and I, especially when I was young. We must have had good times together, too. But the negative memories overshadowed them like storm clouds blot out the sun. The anger hurt. The regret hurt. But most of all, her death still hurt. I didn't want to plumb these depths in front of a stranger.

My father's loss I felt keenly, too. But my relationship with him was solid and stable; I figured this would let me stay composed, no matter what the itako said, the better for me to mentally record the proceedings. Yes, my father made the most sense.

"My mother," I found myself saying.

Something about Také-san must have drawn the response out of me. Itako are mediums, but more to the point, their work is helping survivors come to terms with the loss of their loved ones. That is what itako have done for centuries. That is Také-san's lifework. Grief is like a tunnel, long and dark. If anyone could lead me out of there, maybe it was her. Even though we'd spoken only briefly, something made me feel that she might have the power to facilitate that kind of reconciliation.

Every itako has their own style, inherited from their master, and changed in various ways to suit their own personalities. In order for Také-san to make contact with a deceased person's soul, she told me, she needed to memorize their name, their address, and their date of death, along with the name of the requester and their relationship to the deceased. Because of her age she was quite hard of hearing, and I had to enunciate these words, over and over, until she could recite them herself by heart.

"What is the family name of the person you wish to contact?" she began.

"Yoda."

"Noda."

"No, Yoda."

"Huh?"

"Ya, yu, yo . . . Yoda," I prompted, using the Japanese syllabary.

"Ah, *Yoda*," she said with a little laugh that caused me to giggle, too.

This repeated with the address, and again with my name, her chuckling at her poor hearing and me along with her. It took about ten minutes, and it was hard repeating things like the date of my mother's death aloud at first. But the banter reminded me of afternoons spent with my great-aunt long ago, who took me under her wing like the grandmother I'd never known. We would talk and laugh together just like this. The sense of familiarity only increased when, at one point in the midst of the memorization, Také-san removed two old-fashioned brown sugar candies from the altar's drawer, unwrapping one for herself and offering the other to me.

Once she was satisfied that she had committed the necessary information to memory, she turned to face the altar and rang the Buddhist bell several times in quick succession. Then, even before the resonations had time to die down, she took up her rosary and began to chant. When she moved, the rosary jangled, laden with bone and coin, and the sound of the smooth beads brushing between her palms punctuated the delivery of her incantation.

It began with a recitation of the information I'd given her. Then she began requesting assistance from all sorts of spiritual beings. Kami. Buddhist deities like Lord Enma, the judge of the underworld. Other figures from folklore, said to populate the realm of the dead. Although she never physically moved, it felt as though she were making a pilgrimage to the underworld, building a map of its spiritual terrain, identifying a trail that she might use to navigate there and back to the world of the living.

Soon the invocations gave way to the description of a procession, "led by the thirteen Buddhas," with "Fudo Myo'o," Acala the Implacable, "lighting the way," accompanied by "Shakamuni, whose lotus flowers carry a beautiful fragrance," and on the list continued, Také-san asking them to guide my mother's soul across the River Sanzu for a brief visit to the world of the living. "Descend, descend," she chanted, inviting my mother's spirit into herself. "This is a kuyo," she said, "a remembrance, a request, from your daughter, Yoko."

"Hiroko," I corrected.

". . . From your daughter, Hiroko."

The mistakes didn't bother me. It was apparent at a glance how engaged Také-san was in her efforts. She repeated my mother's name over and over, so many times that I began to wonder if she was having trouble "locating" her soul. Or was it that my mother didn't want to see me?

The chanting continued. Také-san's head nodded deeply again and again, cropped white hair bobbing as she focused her lifetime of experience channeling spirits, for me and my mother. The sight filled me with appreciation. Honestly, it could have ended there and I would have been satisfied, having seen this ancient ritual performed for my benefit.

But suddenly, her voice changed, or rather her cadence did, shifting from chanting to talking. This was my "mother" speaking through Také-san, saying, now, how delighted she was to hear my voice.

She spoke of the sadness she felt at death taking her away, how painful it was not being able to spend more time living with the rest of us. How the sorrow made her restless and she borrowed forms from time to time, a butterfly here, a raven there, aching to say, "I am with you, beside you, protecting you," but death stripped her of her voice, for no matter how powerful their emotion, a soul's words can never reach the ears of the living. Not a day since her death had passed unmarked by tears, but today, today, she heard her daughter's voice beckon, through the itako, to exchange a few words, freed at last to say what she wanted to say.

"It's like a dream," said my "mother."

The monologue lasted about fifty minutes. There was a pattern to it, with Také-san repeating how grateful my mother was, how happy she was to see me, how she would never leave my side. There was little in the way of specifics. I wouldn't argue back if someone pointed out that this reading could well have applied to anyone who'd lost their mother—well, perhaps save that comment about the raven, and then an offhand remark that she wanted me to "enjoy wearing my kimono." But when all was said and done, I realized that the itako's ability to talk to the dead wasn't really a question of true or false, real or not, belief or disbelief. This was a form of grief care, ritualized. A balm for sadness.

In the *Kojiki*, those *Records of Ancient Matters*, kami cry, just like we do when we're sad. But when Izanaki wailed in grief over the loss of his beloved Izanami, his tears turned into kami themselves when they hit the earth. We shed tears throughout our lives, but those we shed out of grief take the most out of us. Did the itako conjure my mother for me? Was it real? I didn't care. My mother was gone forever beyond my reach. That was reality, cold and hard.

But this does not devalue what the itako did for me, as a mourner. For as it turned out, she lifted the veil of negativity concealing our good memories. Perhaps lulled by the rhythmic chanting, I found myself reliving these moments even as the ritual was unfolding, moments long forgotten.

I am a child and we are picking fresh strawberries from a field in the neighborhood.

Now we are pressing wildflowers that we'd found growing around the house.

I am older now, a teen, almost adult. "You're different from the others, Hiroko," she says one day, out of the

*blue. What prompted this? I have no idea. I ask what
she means. "Aishiteiru kara"*—Because I love you.

I hadn't said anything back, hadn't known what to say
back. I was still too young. Why couldn't I respond? I know
from long experience in the US how frequently people say
"I love you" to one another. But we tend to express feelings
differently in Japan. "Aishiteiru" means "I love you," but it
conveys deep and serious feelings, formal and direct, so it is
more commonly used in writing than in speech. I can practically count the number of times I've heard it said. One of
them is the above. Americans vocalize. Japanese tend to
sense, to intuit our intimates' feelings and emotions. Or
that's the ideal.

Don't get me wrong—it isn't that Japanese never express their love for one another verbally. But we express it
in context. I wouldn't realize this until I grew much older.
One way is by saying "arigato." It means "thank you," but
depending on the context, it can carry all the impact of an
English-language "I love you."

Parents teach children to say "thank you" when someone
does them a favor. This is basic etiquette. But as one grows
older, the meanings of those thank-yous grow. They deepen
and widen. What was once casual and reflexive evolves into
something deeper, expressions of affection and gratitude for
someone, or something, that you hold dear.

Gratitude is love. If I could turn the clock back, I know
what I would say back to her: *Thanks, Mom.* The itako made
me realize that. She swept the cobwebs and dust from a
jewel buried deep within me. My mother loved me. She
even said it aloud. I am grateful for that. I am here, thanks
to her. She gave me everything. My anger was real, but these

other things were just as real and true. These memories are why I was wiping tears from my eyes at the end.

....

AFTER THE SESSION, WE RECONVENED IN THE LIVING ROOM for another cup of tea. As we sipped, I took Také-san's hand in mine again.

I thanked her for conducting the ritual. Then I asked her where she thought the underworld might lie, and what it would be like. She interacted with the dead on a daily basis, and had ever since she was young. I was curious about this sightless woman's vision of the world of the dead. But her answer was short and simple.

"I have no idea!" she said with a laugh. "I haven't died yet."

This threw me for a moment. So I changed direction. "Which kami speaks deepest to you?"

"Oh, there are so many," she said. "Too many to choose any one. Which do *you* pray to?"

"I like them all," I laughed. "I pray to everyone."

She smiled and gripped my hand a little tighter. Then she moved her face closer, as though telling me a secret. "There are many kami and hotoke. We both know this. But the truth is, the most important ones of all are the kami of our ancestors. Our family."

When I was six, I'd used a shoebox and a paper flower to make contact with my family in the great beyond. Také-san did the same with her own heart. The beyond lay within her mind. It reminded me that the things we take as holy ground, the shrines and temples and everything else, are just tools. Beautiful tools, but tools nonetheless. True spirituality lays within our hearts and minds. I closed my eyes for a moment, imagining myself at the desk before the altar.

I thought of the universe, vast in its scope, dotted with countless lights of varying sizes and colors. Those were the spirits, and they were shining all around me. When I opened my eyes I could still feel them in my heart.

I told her I had just lost my father, too, and missed him very much. She told me that she lost her father when she was just nineteen. He had worked in the kilns, making charcoal. He had asthma. One day, she noticed he was coming home coughing more than usual. He didn't last very long after that.

"Now I'm past ninety, and I've lived far longer than my father did," she said. "You are like a daughter to me. I want you to live. Live a long and happy life." The words echoed those of my "mother" during the session. When I met the last itako, I expected to talk about death. But I was wrong. The ritual, our conversations before and after—all of it was about how to live. She made that clear, over and over again, in all sorts of ways, during the ritual and after. *Live your life to the fullest. Enjoy your life. Life is full of ups and downs, but when you're feeling low, just remember I'm right there with you.* An itako deals in death so that we find the strength to go on living.

It made me remember a story. I don't know if someone told me this or if I read it somewhere. But it said that when a baby is quickened, they hold their whole life in their hands. When they are born, they release it out into the world. And they spend the rest of their life collecting it. That is what it means to lead a fulfilling life, and it starts from the moment we draw breath on our own. I don't remember what the first thing I collected was. I don't think any of us do. But I suspect I gripped my parents' hands, wrapping my tiny fingers around theirs, a greeting and recognition of my first true guardian angels. I believe that is why I enjoyed walking up that long staircase to Konpira-gu on a toddler's stubborn, unsteady feet. I walked because I trusted in the hands that were holding mine. We were collecting the moments of our lives, me of them and them of me. Because they were always there for me, and always will be.

....

MY FATHER WOULD ASK ME WHAT I WAS WORKING ON, FROM time to time. He had been an entrepreneur and was always curious about my company's clients and projects. He was born in rural Nagano in 1933, the youngest son of nine children. There wasn't enough money for college, and the village was too small to satisfy an ambitious young man like him. He moved to Tokyo, with nothing but a small bag of clothes, and found a job. There were no bullet trains back then, and it took eight hours from Nagano to Tokyo Station. He laughed when I remarked that he could get most of the way to Los Angeles from Tokyo in that amount of time today. He worked for other people at first, then went independent, founding a car-leasing company the same year I was born. He was successful by any measure, but always harbored a certain insecurity about his lack of a college education. He knew there was nothing shameful about it. But it was a sticking point when he dealt with those who cared about that sort of thing. He swore that he would give a good education to his children, and he did.

The last time he asked about my work was on a February morning in the midst of the pandemic. He said he didn't feel well, and was getting ready to take a nap. After he lay down, I sat on a corner of his bed chatting, watching the tsubaki camellia he had planted in the garden outside long ago, now in full crimson bloom.

I was already writing, but it wasn't something I was comfortable speaking about then. Even still, something compelled me to bring it up. Still, I struggled to find the words to explain what I was trying to do in a way he might understand.

"I'm a half century old now," I said with a laugh. "It's time to try something new. I'm writing."

"Oh? What about?"

It was about the spirituality of Japan, I wanted to say. It sounded like religion when I put it that way, but it wasn't, not really. But neither was it not about these things. So many of us think of ourselves as secular, but we aren't as a people, not really. People abroad define themselves by their faiths, but we Japanese live our entire lives in the space between *believe* and *not-believe*. Take the word *kami*. Theoretically, it's Shinto. But that isn't necessarily how it's used in daily speech and life. When we say kami, in general, we aren't inevitably or even commonly indicating Shinto in particular. That mirrors the old animist traditions, the eight million kami of yore, which included all sorts of deities and spirits and even spooks, everything and anything the human mind can imagine. Shinto, Buddhist, folkloric, regional, domestic, foreign—it didn't matter. Even many Buddhist terms have shifted into this soft, welcoming nether realm. Buddhist deities are called hotoke, but in vernacular speech, *hotoke* is another way of referring to "the dead"—to the point even the police use it as slang for a victim. We are Shinto, but not really; we are Buddhist, but so different in practice from that religious order that filtered in from abroad, way back in the sixth century. Even when we hold Buddhist funerals, the goal is the deeply rooted folk practice of kuyo, to help the deceased rest enough that they might manifest as a kami, as future generations would know them, not from memory as we did but from lineage. My father practiced kuyo through the butsudan at the foot of his bed, where he burned incense for my mother and the spirits of his long-departed parents and relatives, every morning before going about his day. The practice was so intertwined in his life, our lives, that the threads became the fabric of life themselves. Whether we believe or not doesn't matter. We just *do*.

I wanted to say all of this to him, but instead I said, "Shinto."

His eyes widened. And he said something that took me by surprise.

"So you're writing about Japanese culture." I'd underestimated him, it seemed. He continued, "I was pretty good at everything, except writing. You certainly didn't get that from me!"

We laughed at that. But quickly the smile faded. He sighed.

"I'm so weak now," he said. "It's depressing." This wasn't like him. I could sense the sadness in his voice. He wanted to offer some advice, I could tell, but didn't know what to say.

"Do I need to remind you that you gave me an education, in two countries, no less? Japan and America both," I said. "You're my number-one supporter."

My studies are precisely why I was able to write, and in a foreign language. He'd given me that gift, and I was endlessly grateful for it. I told him that he'd planted those seeds long ago, and now they were starting to bloom. I didn't know if they would blossom as vividly as the camellia outside his window. But I had the confidence to try, and that was thanks to him.

He didn't reply to this. Just a wan smile, and I left him to his nap.

It was the last real conversation we had.

Right before we closed the lid of my father's coffin, I took his hand in mine for the very last time. The same hand I had held from the first moments of my life. I looked closely at his palm for a while, then laid it down and placed mine beside. For some reason I'd never done this before. It was the first time I ever compared our hands. The creases in our skin were so alike.

I was grateful that we'd had that conversation before he died, and even more grateful that he'd given me the tools to write these words. But he never knew the full scope of what I had in mind. He was from a different generation, when Japan was in a distant corner of the world, far more closed off as a society than it is today. Now it is a thriving international tourist destination, cities filled with people of all kinds, coming for their own reasons but linked by their interest in my country and its traditions. So while he was right that this book is about "Japanese culture," it is also about so much more. I know that now, from all my travels and experiences and reconnecting with my country's traditions. Through them I learned that this flexible way of looking at the great unknowns is relevant to all of us. It speaks to our connections to one another, our connections to the nature that birthed us, always there, even if we don't think about it, buried in our technological lives, even if we deny it for whatever selfish reasons. It isn't about belief; it's about opening your heart.

....

AS I WRITE THESE WORDS, THE FLOODGATES OF MEMORY open. One in particular stands out, a moment when prayer and play intertwined.

The first time I visited Kotohira-gu was as a toddler. But

the only reason I remember that story is because of a second trip I took with my parents, shortly after my nineteenth birthday.

My sister had gone to study abroad, and the program had placed a student from Denmark in our home by way of exchange. He lived with us for three months while he attended a local high school. One day, about a month after he arrived, my father announced that we were going on a weekend trip to see Himeji Castle, a beautiful fortress located in a picturesque town about three hours from Tokyo by bullet train.

The suggestion came out of the blue, but it made sense. My parents wanted to provide their young charge with a memorable Japanese experience. Himeji Castle is my nation's most famous, renowned as the most beautiful in all of Japan. The popular nickname Shirasagi-jo, or "white heron castle," telegraphed its splendor. The main keep, a fortified tower standing 150 feet high, was painted in dazzling white and topped with intricately arching roofwork. Viewed from below, the structure resembled a majestic bird spreading its wings to take flight over the city that it had protected for eight centuries.

We strolled the castle inside and out, exploring its ramparts and moats, its gorgeous interior. It wasn't until we were at the very top of the keep, gazing out over the peaceful city below, that I thought to ask my mother where we were spending the night. Here came another surprise: We weren't staying here at all but catching the train to Kagawa Prefecture, two hours distant. We would find a place to stay when we got there, added my father.

Kagawa is located on the northeast corner of Shikoku, one of the four major islands of Japan. It lies across the Seto

Inland Sea, as we called the body of water separating the main island of Honshu from the islands of Shikoku and Kyushu. Our exchange student was overjoyed, as was I, for a journey over the Inland Sea sounded incredibly exotic to a Tokyo girl like me. We were practically jumping in excitement at this unexpected new adventure to a place I'd only read about, never visited.

Or so I thought. But I'm getting ahead of myself.

First we crossed the sea by train across the Great Seto Bridge. It stretched eight miles over beautiful but treacherous waters, and had taken decades to complete. It had opened only a few years before. It was made of numerous spans bridging a series of tiny islands between Honshu and Shikoku, and crossing it felt a little like you were a stone skipping across the surface of the sea.

In Kagawa we hailed a taxi, and my father directed the driver to take us to the best ryokan in the area. He obliged, dropping us off at one a short drive away. It certainly didn't look like the best inn. In fact, it looked quite old and run-down. My father protested, but the cabbie insisted this was the best place in town. My father's mood darkened even further after we saw the shabby state of our rooms. Neither the exchange student nor I minded, but my father fumed at not being able to deliver the best.

It wasn't until we sat down to dinner that we realized what the taxi driver had meant. Whatever this place lacked in ambience, it more than made up for with the dining room. Waitresses dressed in cherry-blossom-pink kimono brought out a series of ocean delights the likes of which I'd never seen. A moriawase selection of sashimi made from local catch, arrayed on a wooden boat that evoked the fisherfolk who'd brought it to the docks hours before. Delicate arrangements of tempura, so expertly prepared that it made the deep-fried morsels seem almost light. Wakame sea-weed, bright green, so fresh it felt as though it had been plucked directly from the sea. Grilled fish that made your mouth water by sight.

As I write, more memories flood back. We were brought a basket of exceptionally large botan ebi shrimp, so plump and fresh that they looked still alive to my eyes. I always loved shrimp, but I was so busy with the smorgasbord of dishes in front of me that I wasn't paying attention. My mother, seemingly worried I'd miss out on what she knew was a favorite dish, peeled one and handed it to me.

"I'm coming of age next year," I laughed, "and still need my mother to peel my shrimp!" She laughed, too. I still remember that shrimp, soft and sweet and delicate, practically melting in my mouth. Somehow, that one moment symbolized the whole evening to me.

It reminds me that Japanese don't call seafood "seafood" as such. Instead, we use a more poetic term: "umi no sachi"—"happiness from the sea." And our grand course wasn't limited to seafood. There were delicious dishes made from fresh harvests of vegetables. We call foods harvested from the land "yama no sachi"—"happiness from the mountains." They come from different worlds, but on the tabletop they combine into more than the sum of their parts.

The sashimi slices were served nestled on a bed of delicately shredded daikon radish. It was garnished with shiso leaves and chrysanthemum blossoms. And, of course, pungent horseradish, made from grating the roots of the wasabi plant. All of it atop a vessel shaped like a boat. Delights from land and sea, coming together in harmony like the Seven Gods of Happiness aboard their treasure ship.

After we sat down, and before we picked up our chopsticks, we said "itadakimasu" together, just like we always did every time we ate together. And while I truly did "receive with gratitude," as the word literally means, I was receiving something much more than food: the happiness of being together with family, so enveloping it was inexpressible. Until now.

The next morning, we set out for Kotohira-gu. As we stood at the bottom of that long stone staircase, contemplating the climb, my father delivered yet another surprise.

"This isn't your first time here, you know," he said. "We brought you here when you were a toddler. And you even walked these steps on your own two feet . . ."

It took us quite some time to make it to the shrine at the top. Part of this was because we stopped for sweet dango with green tea midway up. But it was mainly because my Dane host-brother and I poked our heads into every souvenir shop along the way—and there were a lot of them. Whenever one of us would find something funny or interesting, we'd call out to share our excitement with the others. An oversize paper fan caught my fancy. Paper fans are normally around a foot long, handle and paper paddle included. This one was laughably huge—easily two and half feet tall, bright red, and festooned with a hand-inked character reading *matsuri*, or "festival." For some reason this made me laugh, so much so that my mother actually bought it for me.

I must have looked silly climbing those stairs carrying a fan almost half my height. In fact, I know I did, because my host-brother kept giggling every time he looked over and saw me carrying the thing. "I can't believe she actually bought you that," he laughed. I actually agreed with him. But buy it my mother had, because she saw how much fun I was having. She obviously wanted to let me enjoy the moment.

As we approached the prayer hall at the top of the steps, I put the fan gently on the ground and turned to my parents.

"If Kotohira-gu was the first shrine that I visited in my life, I'd better tell the kami-sama that little baby has grown up. I need to thank them for that!"

And then we all prayed together.

For many years I'd mourned not being able to celebrate my coming of age, as my sister had, in her beautiful furisode. But as I write these words, I finally realize that doesn't mean I was deprived. I simply had a different sort of celebration. A celebration together with my mother and father and the kami whom I'd first greeted on my tiny feet, almost two decades before. I was simply too young to have seen it then. I am grateful I lived long enough to see it now.

....

EVERYTHING IS PERSPECTIVE.

We live in a world divided, barraged by demands for our attention and time, our allegiance and faith. The unfathomable complexity of life, with all its contradictions and paradoxes and unpredictability, all its high points and low points, all its joy and sorrow, is precisely what fuels a demand for such black-and-white solutions. But our world is not so easily tamed by the categorizations of the human mind. We live in a universe of dynamic contrasts and contradictions and differences, on scales ranging from the unfathomably large to the indescribably tiny and everything between. Terrain to culture, skin tone to orientation. And these are just the differences we can see. Reality is far more varied and vibrant than the human mind can imagine.

That's what makes the "yaoyorozu-no-kami"—eight million kami—so important. I'd thought of this as a Shinto term, because it originated there. But I was wrong. It's so much bigger than that. The word *kami* may be Japanese, but the kami themselves aren't, not really. They are the things that surround us, the avatars of what we can see and imagine, and those things we can't or won't.

Their uncountable multitude reminds us that there is always space for something new and different. As I write this, my father's voice is echoing in my head. "Differences are good. If you can respect them, they are the keys to making bigger and better things."

It reminds us that spirituality is ours to take hold of, or to let go; ours to belong in, or choose not to; ours to believe in, or not; ours to interact with through an organized religion, or through a more personal and playful lens. Because there are as many ways to cultivate spirituality as there are people. Each of us carries our own universe in our minds. But this doesn't mean we are the center of the universe. Like the Seven Gods of Happiness, we are all bound together on this treasure ship called Earth. We would do well to take a page from their example.

I can feel the kami. When a gentle breeze rustles my hair. When the sunlight warms my skin. When the birds trill and the ravens watch me with eyes of obsidian. When I feel these things, I can feel them.

You don't need a shrine to feel these things. You don't need permission. You just need to open your heart enough to hear the "voices." Because I, you, me, all of us, are surrounded by the kami, eight million of them and more, the sun, the earth, our ancestors and family. When I think about that, I'm never alone. And neither are you. Life is full of ups and downs, soaring highs and painful lows. But no matter how hard things get, we don't have to go through them alone. There are so many different ways to heal. There are so many different ways to happiness.

Epilogue

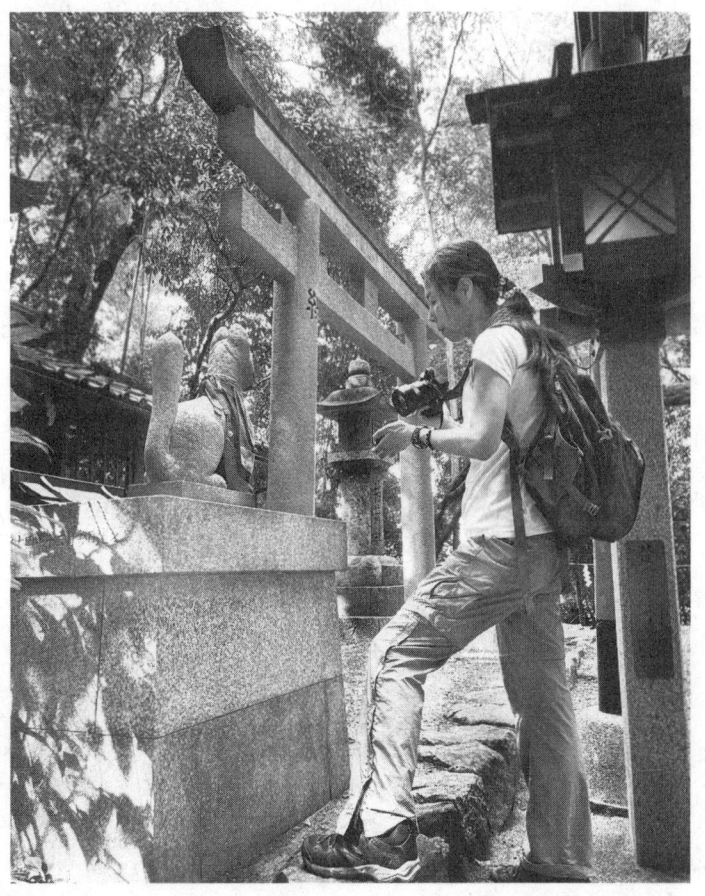

Once a month or so, my husband and I go over to my old childhood home, now occupied by my sister and her family, for an early dinner. She and I generally do the cooking, and on one particular early-summer day, the two of us decided that we were in the mood for karé raisu—Japanese-style curry rice. It's a hearty, aromatic, gravy-like stew, filled with meat and vegetables, that is ladled over steaming white rice. It's one of my country's favorite dishes, a classic comfort food, so popular that it is often referred to as a national dish.

Everyone has their own preferences: Sweet or spicy? Mild or hot? Meat- or vegetable-based? Thick or soupy? But my sister and I decided to go for what might be called the basic style that day, because my tween niece had taken an interest in cooking and wanted to learn how to make it for herself. We chose a straightforward selection of ingredients: onions, carrots, potatoes, and chunks of beef, all of which would be mixed with a block of premade roux. (Curry is so popular here that competing brands of roux can sometimes fill entire aisles of supermarkets.) This was the same style of curry that my mother had taught my sister and me to make, many years ago. Now it was our turn to pass it down to the next generation.

First, the three of us began slicing the vegetables and beef into bite-size chunks. We tossed them into a pot and stir-fried them for a bit, then added water and simmered until tender. Next we added the block of roux. As it dissolved into the mix, the unmistakable aroma of Japanese curry instantly filled the room, sweet and spicy, pungent and inviting. While this fragrant broth stewed, we began prepping the rice.

We always talk a lot while we cook. We talk a lot anyway, but there's something about focusing on a simple, repetitive task with your hands that really makes you want to chat. As my sister and I caught up over happenings since the last gathering, the topic of my writing came up. My niece asked about the differences between Japan and America. I mentioned that America was home to a much larger population of Christians than Japan, and what that meant in daily life and holidays. One particular point really took her by surprise.

"Wait," said my niece in shock. "Christians don't have butsudan?"

I smiled. Not at her reaction but because it reminded me of my own first encounters with cultural and spiritual differences, so many years ago. I knew where her surprise came from. She'd grown up in a home with a butsudan altar. She'd never known a life without one. I smiled because she made me feel as though I were coming full circle.

My niece was born a year after our mother's passing, when the family was still grieving. A little ray of sunshine in that darkness. She grew up watching her parents, her grandfather, and my husband and me offering incense, water, flowers, and sweets at the butsudan as we prayed for the grandmother whom she'd never know, as I hadn't known mine. When she grew big enough to understand, her parents guided her in joining this ritual, and she would put her palms together, too.

The butsudan wasn't just for her grandmother. It was an exquisitely finished box of wood about a foot and a half on a side, sitting beneath a shelf. On it were arranged family photos, of grandparents and great-grandparents who had long since departed our world. My mother's was the most recent face among them. A few years later, she would be joined by a photo of my father, and then one of my brother-in-law's father, too.

My niece saw this in her home, and I'm sure she saw

similar things in the homes of her friends. The butsudan is so quotidian, so much a part of daily life, that she didn't think it religious at all. It was simply a tool for maintaining a connection with the departed. That's why she took it for granted that everyone might have one. Even Christians. Which is why I replied:

"I know what you mean. For us, a butsudan is simply a way for communicating with people who are gone. Many people don't even think of them in religious terms. But a Christian would almost certainly see it as a religious object, a Buddhist one in particular." Her brow furrowed; I could tell, she was even more confused.

"I know, I know," I continued. "We don't identify as Buddhist. Yet we have a Buddhist altar in the house. It's a little complicated, but you don't have to understand the details right now. All you need to know is that we Japanese are very flexible when it comes to spirituality."

As if on cue, the rice cooker beeped, signaling that the rice was done. My sister popped the lid and began scooping our portions of rice into the serving dishes. But she must have scooped a little too hard, for a chunk of rice bounced off one dish and landed in the sink with a thud. We all stopped for a moment and peered at the forlorn little mound.

"My teacher said there are seven kami in every grain of rice," remarked my niece.

"Well, this is even more of a disaster, then," laughed my sister.

Smiling, we put our palms together, a quick prayer for the fallen rice. None of us took this all that seriously—it was a routine cooking spill in the kitchen. But neither did we mean it derisively, either.

Then we got back to work. As we busied ourselves plating the curry, I asked out of curiosity:

"Did your teacher tell you which kami were in the rice?"

"Nope." My niece shrugged. This elicited another laugh. But, you know, that's Japanese spirituality for you. There are eight million kami, after all; the details don't matter. All that does is knowing the kami are out there. They remind us what's important. Rice connects us: the farmers who made it, the family we are sharing it with, the nutrition it gives us to stay healthy. And, of course, the pleasure of eating it.

Rice is so fundamental to Japanese culture that it is a synonym for the word *food*. When we say we want to eat, we say we want "gohan," which literally means "a bowl of rice," but colloquially it simply means "food." From virtually the moment we are able to raise chopsticks and feed ourselves, whether at home or school, we are always told: *Finish your gohan. Don't leave even a grain of rice behind.*

The kami teach us to be thankful, grateful, humble. Recognizing them helps us appreciate the things around us, big and small. If that isn't the foundation of happiness, I don't know what is.

....

OVER THE YEARS, PEOPLE WHO THINK ABOUT THESE SORTS of things have come up with many different ways of referring to Japan's patchwork of religious traditions. *Shinbutsu shugo* (the fusion of kami and bodhisattvas) is the most official-sounding one. More casually, you'll hear even religious scholars using adjectives like *zatta* (jumbled up). And then there's "gotta-ni," which means "hodgepodge," a simple but hearty stew of influences.

While I was making dinner together with my sister and niece, talking about butsudan and kami, I started to think that curry might be an even more apt, and fun, metaphor for

Japanese spirituality. This might sound silly. It made me laugh when I first thought it up. But I am also completely serious. I believe that Japanese karé, not "curry"—or rather the way it is most often eaten in Japan, as karé raisu—is actually the perfect metaphor for our three major belief systems of Shinto, Buddhism, and Shugendo. And the ways we cook and serve it symbolize how average folks interact with those spiritual traditions. So let me say it again.

Japanese spirituality is like a nice, steaming bowl of karé raisu.

That fragrant sauce reminds me of Japan's approach to Buddhism. Similar to how Japan imported Buddhism from India by way of China in the seventh century, Japan imported karé from India by way of the British sailors who first introduced it to our shores in the late nineteenth century. Over the century and a half since, we "localized" it from an exotic foreign import into a meal uniquely suited to our particular tastes. Indian curries are known for their spiciness. Japanese karé tends to be sweet and mild, which is why it is a favorite of children. Back then, it was a dish for the few worldly enough to have interactions with foreigners. In this early incarnation, the dish was known as raisu karé, or rice curry.

The beef reminds me of Christianity, for it is a contribution from the Christian nations that began doing business with us after our ports opened to the world. For more than a millennium, since the introduction of Buddhism to Japan, the consumption of game and livestock had been seen as taboo. In fact, it was legally prohibited by a long-standing imperial decree. But after the opening of the ports, the Meiji government, eager to mimic the behavior of successful Western nations, repealed the order. The biggest importers of cattle into Japan at the time were Americans, so into Japan's Indian-inspired British curry went American beef.

Raisu karé remained a luxury until the 1960s, when a new evolution of the dish appeared: prepackaged karé roux, sold at supermarkets for a very reasonable price. Now, instead of having to cook karé from scratch, you could use a block of roux to jump-start the process and make a quick, satisfying meal for your whole family. Instant roux sparked a society-wide karé boom. Here, too, we see parallels to Buddhism, as a new way of thinking and living percolated down from the elites to the masses, from the rice curry of the nineteenth-century upper crust to the karé raisu upon which successive postwar generations of children were raised.

The rice represents Shinto. *Records of Ancient Matters* and *Chronicles of Japan* refer to our land as "toyoashihara-no-mizuho-no-kuni"—"a country rich in water, with abundant rice." Rice is more than food; it is life itself, which is why it and rice wine are offered in Shinto rituals, expressing the bonds between us and the earth, between people and the eight million kami. A bowl of karé raisu is constructed from a generous ladle of that thick stew brimming with foreign influences, but it sits atop a sturdy, tasty foundation of rice from Japan.

And the metaphor deepens: You can adjust your karé rice however you like. There is no such thing as a karé rice identitarian or fundamentalist! More rice than sauce, or vice versa? It's all up to you—an echo of the way so many Japanese adjust their own spiritual traditions. The karé sauce is the "Buddhism" to rice's "Shinto," served up invitingly on a single plate, the flavors mixing so harmoniously that the combination has emerged as a national favorite and a new kind of culinary tradition.

I said there were two elements to karé raisu, but there's actually a third, and that is *where* you eat it. And this is how I think karé raisu resembles yet another Japanese spiritual tradition: Shugendo.

Curry is served in restaurants and homes, of course. But whenever people gather outdoors, you'll inevitably find curry there, too. In elementary school, our teachers took the class on a field trip to a campground. There were about forty kids in all. The teachers split us into six smaller groups and helped each group of students work together to cook their own lunch—which was, you guessed it: karé raisu.

Cooking and eating outdoors is a kind of dance with nature. The Shugendo yamambushi treat mountains as spiritual realms, places where the logic and order of towns and human settlements doesn't necessarily apply. It's the same way with karé rice outdoors. Everything you take for granted in a modern kitchen goes out the window. There's no electricity or gas, so there's no stovetop. Often you need to gather rocks to make a firepit, then kindling to start a fire, and carefully tend it, too.

Gathering kindling was my assigned task on that long-ago field trip. My teacher told me to gather different sizes of wood. I asked her why, and she told me "Every fire starts small, just like a baby," she told me. "And you need to feed it to grow. Little sticks to get started, bigger to keep it going." She also told me to fetch a bucket of water, because fire could be dangerous. These were some of the first lessons I learned about living outdoors, and I owe them to karé raisu.

Even after I grew up, I noticed that karé remains the go-to food for camp cookouts, especially in big groups. Since we need to make so much food, we all divide up the task of prepping the vegetables and other ingredients. This makes things easier, but it also makes the cutting boards stages for individuality. Karé rice is so popular that everyone has their own preferences, and it's fun to see the differences in how everyone, say, chops onions: Thinly sliced? Diced? Big chunks? The flexibility of karé, its ability to take whatever we throw into it, mirrors the flexibility of our spirituality. And even the ingredients differ from person to person. Some prefer to add corn or pumpkin for a sweeter taste; others like mixing in eggplant for the distinct texture it imparts. Once a friend dumped in a handful of bamboo shoots she harvested from a grove in her neighborhood. When it comes to karé, and particularly camp-style karé, there's never really any wrong way. There's always room for a new ingredient—just like there's always room for a new kami among the eight million.

The sky, grass, trees, the breeze, everything around us also combines into a spice more important than any single ingredient: gratitude. Our combined work and effort make that meal taste all the better. Add to the gratitude a dash of happiness, a pinch of friendship, a spoonful of camaraderie. We have a saying in Japanese, "Onaji kama no meshi wo kuu," which literally means "to eat out of the same pot." It means sharing food brings us closer—all of us. Young and old, male and female, Japanese and non-Japanese. When we dip into the same pot, we become friends. And when the party's over, all of us cooperate to clean up the area. We tear old newspaper into strips to wipe down the pots and plates before washing them, to save water. We put all of our trash into garbage bags that we carry out with us. We were only "borrowing" the space from the mountains. It's our responsibility to ensure it stays how it was when we found it.

So there's all that. But most of all, karé raisu is fun to

share. I like to think the same is true for Japan's spiritual traditions as well.

....

IN 1909, A WRITER BY THE NAME OF KAKUZO OKAKURA PUB-lished *The Book of Tea*, one of the very first English-language books on the topic of Japanese spiritual traditions, authored by a native Japanese. It was a guide to the tea ceremony, but it was also something more. "Strangely enough humanity has so far met in the tea-cup," he wrote, describing the beverage as one of the few Asian traditions that "commands universal esteem." The slim but bold volume won Okakura many fans in New York's high society because it explained the concepts of Taoism, "Zennism" (as he called Zen Buddhism), and other philosophies to the world—all through the lens of tea.

I see karé raisu, Japanese curry rice, in much the same way—imported, transformed, and exported again, to the delight and fascination of outsiders. *The New York Times* even included a Japanese katsu curry dish, which is karé on rice with tonkatsu pork cutlets, as one of the "23 of the Best American Dishes of 2023"—showing just how far karé raisu has come. It speaks to how "Japanese things" aren't necessarily only for the Japanese anymore. And how there's really no fixed definition of "Japanese things" anyway, because our traditions change as we share them with the outside world.

Here's a perfect example. You may recall me writing about bon-odori, the bon dances that communities all over Japan hold to celebrate the season of their ancestors' spirits returning to our world in late summer. I'd long fallen out of the habit of going to bon dances. But in the summer of 2024, I decided to give it a try again. The place I chose is called Nakano. It is famed as one of Tokyo's subcultural spots because it is home to a shopping center specializing in all sorts of anime, manga, and other fun stuff. But that wasn't why I picked it. Nakano is a larger, more urban neighborhood than my own, and I simply wanted to see what a modern bon-odori might look like. And so for the first time in thirty or more years, I put on my festival wear—my yukata robe and sandals—and headed out for some fun.

The Nakano bon-odori was *way* different from the festivals I remembered from my youth. The first thing I noticed was there weren't many vendor stalls, and none of them had toys or games. They sold beer and shaved ice, but no playthings. This wasn't for any lack of children. Perhaps it is because kids are more interested in video games and apps these days, or perhaps because toys seem less a treat when you can get them anytime you want, as you can from the city's now ubiquitous capsule toy vending machines. And the food stalls were fun but didn't feel as necessary—the festivities were in an urban park, surrounded by convenience stores, fast-food shops, and cafés. Festivalgoers could simply pop in to any one without lining up. It was undeniably convenient, but it felt different from the local festivals I remembered.

Then there was the dancing. Rather than a large scaffold of the type you see in neighborhood festivals, Nakano's featured a slightly raised platform, maybe three feet high, on top of which were four professional (or at least well practiced) bon-odori dancers. Everyone else danced around this platform while watching the "pros" for cues as to hand and foot motions. The music wafted over from the speakers of a mega-size sound system erected on a stage nearby.

They played classics from time to time, but most were remixes, fast and fun—*really* fast and fun. Many bon-odori songs, even classics, are based on anime themes or pop songs, so the selections weren't shocking. But the moves were! In contrast to the stately shuffle of traditional bon dance, these had many steps forward, backward, sideways, with a lot of spinning, turning, and jumping. Many participants wore yukata, but the dances felt modern, even cutting-edge. I started laughing as I tried to keep up: *What is this? Exercise class?*

Between dances, the stage would come to life. At one point, a band began playing electrified bon music—live. This was something you simply didn't see or hear at local festivals, which relied on recordings. The crowd turned from the dance platform to the stage, dancing on the spot, like a concert. Some wore Hello Kitty–esque bows on their head, or flashing rings, both illuminated by multicolored LEDs. (Vendors worked the crowd selling each for a hundred yen, less than a dollar.) All the flashing lights and synchronized moves reminded me less of obon than ota-gei, the term for the hyperfans of idol singers waving colored light sticks in unison at a concert. But the biggest surprise was yet to come: a middle-aged lady in yukata, who wouldn't have looked out of place at any local festival, took center stage. Then she led the crowd in a traditional bon-odori routine—to the accompaniment of Jon Bon Jovi's "Livin' on a Prayer"!

Later I learned that playing Bon Jovi has become a "thing" for Nakano's bon-odori festival. His name has "Bon" in it, after all, and in a super pop-conscious place like Nakano, it was probably only a matter of time before someone made the connection. The organizers have been doing it for quite a few years now, and it has grown so popular that it attracted the attention of the man himself. "It is great to know that 'Livin' on a Prayer' has been loved and used for bon-odori for many years," said Bon Jovi in a 2024 video message. "Have fun dancing this summer, too!"

All of this reminds me of how prayer and play intertwine in Japanese spirituality. From my experience in the West, prayer is a serious and even solemn thing. The concept of playful spirituality might even seem a little sacrilegious there. But not here. In Japan, spiritual traditions coexist with modern secular culture in all sorts of ways, such as the vibrant shopping streets leading to many Buddhist temples. Bon-odori is another great example. And the Bon Jovi song shows how this thinking goes beyond borders.

After the Nakano party, as we walked home from our local train station, my husband and I heard the drumming of traditional Obon songs. It could mean only one thing: The neighborhood festival was happening, right now! The very one I'd once gone to as a child. We hurried past our house and to the source of the commotion. The festival was much smaller in scale than Nakano's, with a more traditional arrangement. It was being held in a newly renovated bus terminal area, a wide-open space, much better than the cramped locations I remembered from my youth. The songs here were, if anything, even more pop-forward and faster than Nakano's. And the kids were really into it. At times the crowd even ran around the central scaffold! It was so different from in my childhood, but equally raucous and joyous. As I joined them to dance, for the second time that night, I felt as though I was witnessing the passing of a torch between generations.

That's what bon, and Japanese spirituality as a whole, is all about: connection. Between the departed and the living, between old traditions and new trends, between religious and nonreligious, between East and West, and among all of us who participate. I had a thirty-year blank spot in my bon-odori history, but these festivities made me feel as if I hadn't missed a beat.

AS I DANCED, IN THIS PLACE SO NEAR THE SPOT MY MOTHER
took me to my first bon-odori, thoughts of her danced
through my head. As it happened, they played my old childhood favorite, "The 21st Century Dance," for the night's fi-
nale. The familiar tune reminded me again of my childhood,
but that nostalgia was tinged by reminders of how much
time had passed, and how much things had changed. What
had been almost new in my childhood was now fifty-five
years old, and the lyrics were laughably out of date. The line
about "the twenty-first century coming soon" made the
kids giggle and the adults roll their eyes. Yet the vibe remained excited, vibrant, joyous. I found my feet making familiar patterns, patterns I'd picked up as a little girl. As the
crowd circled around the scaffold, it felt as though the clock
were running backward, and as we whirled, it was as
though I was seeing double—myself in the here and now,
and myself decades earlier. Both of us in yukata. One I'd
purchased myself, recently; the other, one sewn by my
mother, years ago.

As we danced together, a new memory unlocked, one
from between these two times of youth and middle age,
from the turn of the millennium in 2001. That was the year
I received an unexpected postcard in the mail. It was from
my parents, and they had written it in 1985. It seemed they'd
visited something called the International Exposition in Tsu-
kuba, and the event offered a "time capsule" for those who
wished to send a message to someone in the future, in that
twenty-first century to come. I'd had no idea they'd done
this until the card arrived at their home and they handed it
to me, sixteen years after they'd posted it. The address was
penned in my father's familiar script; the message, though,
was in my mother's hand, then still strong and clear.

Your mom and dad are at the Exposition.
Your name may not be Yoda when you receive this.
We believe the 21st century will be a wonderful one.

She was right: I'd married in 1999, to the man who was now holding my drink for me outside the dance circle as I made a final turn, just as my mother had held my half-melted cotton candy so long ago. As the memories flooded back, it was easy to imagine her standing next to him, watching her daughter dancing.

I'd always tended to frame my memories with my mother as either "good" or "bad." I still do this, to tell you the truth, because old habits are hard to break. But when I danced, at that moment, I started to think that maybe I shouldn't think in such polarized terms. Memories are memories. Experiences are experiences. All of them equally precious, because they're more than afterimages: They're my life. They're *me*. If I couldn't acknowledge my past, how could I acknowledge myself?

This was a neighborhood festival but it was something more at this moment, a spiritual place, my dancing an offering, a prayer——to the parents who gave me life and the experiences that delivered me to this place at this moment, spinning in my old neighborhood while the earth spun though the cosmos, bringing me to just the right spot, like it had when I triggered the shutter on that raven so many years ago.

If I cried now, the tears wouldn't be of sadness. Nor would they be of joy. They would be of life, the life I'd lived, the lives that supported me, and that I wanted to support in turn. That was my new journey. And this book would be its first step. A record of my travels. Like my great-grandfather's diary from over a century before.

The path ahead wouldn't always be easy. I knew that from experience. But I wouldn't be alone. No matter where I was, the eight million kami would be there for me. As they will for you, too, whether you choose to acknowledge them or never give them a second thought. It's all right.

For spirituality can be found anywhere—high and low and everywhere between, in the seas and mountains, in the forests and fields, in luminous light and enveloping darkness. Even in the foods we eat and the dances we dance. Spirituality isn't an identity; it's the world itself. It's how we live. It is about inclusion, not exclusion. It is about recognition, not rejection. It is about gratitude, respect, and love. It's a way of thinking that can unlock new possibilities, sustain through difficult times, and quietly nourish during unremarkable ones. That is what makes Japan's unique approach so relevant to everyone, even those who haven't been to Japan, even those who may never go.

Records of Ancient Matters calls humans "ao-hito-kusa"—"green-grass people." It reminds us of where we came from, and where we will return. In the end, the earth is our biggest supporter, making it possible for us to take breath and live, giving us the nutrition and encouragement to grow, like our mothers did, like the mother earth does to all of us. The planet is the treasure boat upon which all of us ride, just as the Seven Gods of Happiness ride upon theirs, their camaraderie a lesson for us all.

My book ends here, but all our journeys continue. The eight million kami symbolize the diversity of worldviews in everything around us, and within us. Listen to their voices, for they have much to teach. Gratitude is their gift to us, and it has the power to sustain us through difficult times, whenever and wherever we might be.

Acknowledgments

First, I'd like to thank my husband, Matt Alt, for his support at every possible turn. We've been working together for more than a quarter of a century, first as localizers of others' content, and now as creators of our own. Two independent authors under the same roof! I'm so proud of what we've accomplished together.

I could never forget to thank my agent, Dado Derviskadic, for his passion and expertise helped make my transition to author happen. I will always remember what he told me the night before we sent the proposal for this book to publishers. "Everything is laid out for you. Now all you have to do is follow the path." I was so nervous that I barely slept, but those words really encouraged me and put me at ease.

A big thank-you to my editor, Emi Ikkanda, for her enthusiasm and support. Her feedback at every stage was so richly detailed, and her keen questions expanded my horizons about my own spiritual culture. My book would never have become what it did without her editorial insight.

And to Phoebe Robinson, thank you for welcoming me to Tiny Reparations by sending me a bonsai! That happy little tree, an Okinawan "gajumaru," has been sitting next to my desk as my writing buddy ever since it arrived. Okinawan legend has it that gajumaru trees are homes to yokai that bring good fortune. I believe!

I'd also like to thank Kazuo Kiuchi, Meghan Houser, Shinkichi, and the many others I met along the way for their help. I am blessed to be surrounded by people with amazing talents, deep knowledge, and incredible personal connections. I appreciate each and every one of them, for without their help, I would never have made it this far.

Last but not least, deepest thanks to my family, close and extended, and my parents most of all. Even though you'll never have the chance to read these words, I know you are proud of me. I miss you a lot, and love you forever.

Notes

PROLOGUE

7 **"happiness and unhappiness can't be considered":** "Shinoda Toko ga nokoshita kotoba 'toshi wo torukoto wa atarashii hakken wo erukoto'" ("Toko Shinoda's Words of Wisdom 'As You Age You Discover New Things'"), *Fujin Koron* website, April 2, 2021, accessed September 19, 2024, https://fujinkoron.jp/articles/-/3561?page=5.

7 **"The notion that one's goal in life":** *The Kingdom of Dreams and Madness*, directed by Mami Sunada (Toho, Japan, 2013).

7 **The author Yukio Mishima was even more:** Yukio Mishima, *Sun and Steel* (Tokyo: Kodansha International, 1970), 57.

10 **philosopher Norinaga Motoori defined kami:** "Jitsuwa zennintowa kagiranai 'nihon no kamisama' odoroki noshotai: isshin kyo no sekai towa okiku kotonaru toyo no shiso," *Toyo Keizai Online*, January 18, 2021, accessed September 19, 2024, https://toyokeizai.net/articles/-/403893.

10 **cultural anthropologist Dr. Kazuhiko Komatsu:** Kazuhiko Komatsu, *Yokai-gaku Shinko (New Yokai Studies)* (Tokyo: Shogakukan, 1994), 35.

18 **the building of "a spiritual toolbox":** World Council of Churches, "Johan Galtung: Religions Have Potential for Peace," May 24, 2012, accessed September 19, 2024, https://www.oikoumene.org/news/johan-galtung-religions-have-potential-for-peace.

18   Way back in 1894, the Japanologist Lafcadio Hearn: Lafcadio
      Hearn, *Glimpses of Unfamiliar Japan* (Tokyo: Charles E. Tuttle,
      1976), 386.

19   This is why Western journalists write: Max Fisher and
      Caitlin Dewey, "A Surprising Map of Where the World's
      Atheists Live," *Washington Post*, May 23, 2013.

19   organizations claim almost 180 million followers: Hiroyuki
      Mantani, ed., Shukyo Kanren *Tokei ni Kan Suru Shiryoushu*
      (*Materials Regarding Religious-Related Statistics*) (Tokyo: Agency
      for Cultural Affairs, Government of Japan, 2014), 3, accessed
      August 12, 2024, https://www.bunka.go.jp/tokei_hakusho
      _shuppan/tokeichosa/shumu_kanrentokei/pdf/h26_chosa.pdf

CHAPTER 1:
THE INVISIBLES: SHINTO

41   "The beauty of Ise": Donald Keene, *On Familiar Terms: To
      Japan and Back, a Lifetime Across Cultures* (Tokyo: Kodansha
      International, 2007), 162.

45   Iwao Oba, a professor of Shinto archaeology: Muneaki
      Yoshikawa, *Ganseki wo Shinko Shiteita Nihonjin* (*The Japanese
      Who Worshiped Stone*) (Osaka: U-Time Publishing, 2011), 39.

49   "chill even in the sun": Lafcadio Hearn, *Glimpses of Unfamiliar
      Japan*, vol. 1 (New York: Houghton, Mifflin, 1894), 23.

49   "I reach the altar, gropingly": Hearn, *Glimpses*, 23.

51   "If you ask me, there's nothing better": Haruki Murakami,
      Murakami Asahido (*Murakami's House of the Rising Sun*) (Tokyo:
      Shinchosha, 1987), 190.

CHAPTER 2:
THE HARMONY OF CONFLICT: BUDDHISM

57   Professor D. T. Suzuki, who transmitted Zen: Daisetz T.
      Suzuki, *Zen and Japanese Culture* (Princeton University Press,
      1959), 215.

64 **"true harmony only emerges from conflict":** Kazuaki Kajiwara, *Honda Soichiro no Tetsugaku* ("The Philosophy of Soichiro Honda") (Kyoto: PHP Institute, 2002).

64 **"disharmony the building block of harmony":** Akiomi Hirano, *Taro Okamoto Taiyo no To to Saigo no Tatakai* ("Taro Okamoto's Final Battle for the Tower of the Sun") (Kyoto: PHP Institute, 2009) 125.

72 **In this we were not alone:** "Niwanao Heiwa Zaidan: Nihonjin no shukyo dantai ni tai suru seron chosa; 20 nen kamidana iranai, butsudan iranai katei ga zoka" ("Niwano Peace Foundation: A Survey of Japanese People's Attitudes Towards Religious Groups; Families Who Say They Don't Want Kamidana or Butsudan Increase for 20 Years"), *Kosei Shimbun Digital*, October 10, 2019, https://shimbun.kosei-shuppan.co .jp/news/34925/.

72 **In a 2018 interview, she elaborated:** Rebecca Milner, "How I Get It Done: Organizational Guru Marie Kondo," *The Cut*, March 6, 2018, https://www.thecut.com/2018/03/marie -kondo-lifechanging-magic-tidying-up-interview.html.

72 **Haruki Murakami has written about kamidana:** Haruki Murakami, afterword to F. Scott Fitzgerald, *Gureeto Gyatsubi* (*The Great Gatsby*), trans. Haruki Murakami (Tokyo: Chuokoron-Shinsha, 2006), 327.

82 **In 2024, the Pew Research Center:** Jonathan Evans et al., *Report, June 17, 2024, Religion and Spirituality in East Asian Societies*, "2. Religion as a way of life," Pew Research Center, accessed August 9, 2024, https://www.pewresearch.org /religion/2024/06/17/religion-as-a-way-of-life/#importance -of-religion-around-the-world.

82 **Yet Japan is also home:** *e-Stat: Seifu Sokei no Madoguchi* (*e-Stat: Government Statistics Portal*), accessed August 9, 2024, https:// www.e-stat.go.jp/dbview?sid=0003282942.

82 **By way of comparison, we have "only" 55,000:** Japan Franchise Association website, accessed August 9, 2024, https://www.jfa-fc.or.jp/particle/320.html.

85 As the folklorist Noboru Miyata put it: *Edo no Chiisana Kamigami* (*The Many Little Kami of Edo*) (Japan: Seidosha, 1997), 229.

CHAPTER 3:
MAKING FRIENDS WITH MONSTERS: SHUGENDO

88 "Everyone, at some point in their lives": Nanae Miura, "Oajari Ryojin Shionuma San ni Manabu, Shiawase na Jinsei no Arukikakta" ("Oajari Ryojin Shionuma on How to Live a Happy Life"), *Kappo*, March 9, 2021, retrieved September 1, 2024, https://kappo.machico.mu/articles/4811.

88 "I never visit a shrine for New Year's": Hayao Miyazaki, *Starting Point: 1979–1996*, trans. Beth Cary and Frederik L. Schodt (San Francisco: Viz Media, 2014), 360.

95 "Westerners tend to think of light": Roman Album Extra 69: *Tonari no Totoro* (*My Neighbor Totoro*) (Japan: Tokuma Shoten, 1988), 128.

96 Perhaps this is because "Buddhism and Shinto": Helen Hardacre, *Shinto: A History* (New York: Oxford University Press, 2017), 180.

97 Jesuit missionaries first encountered Shugendo: Linda Zampol D'Ortia, Lucia Dolce, and Ana Fernandes Pinto, "Saints, Sects, and (Holy) Sites: The Jesuit Mapping of Japanese Buddhism, Sixteenth Century," in *Interactions between Rivals: The Christian Mission and Buddhist Sects in Japan (c.1549–c.1647),* ed. Alexandra Curvelo and Angelo Cattaneo (Berlin: Peter Lang, 2021), 78.

97 "In the depths of certain mountains": Carmen Blacker, *The Catalpa Bow: A Study in Shamanistic Practices in Japan* (England: Taylor & Francis, 1999), x.

99 "In a 2007 book, he described": Ryojun Shionuma and Koshu Itabashi, *Omine Sennichi Kaihogyo* (*A Thousand Days Training in Omine*) (Shunjusha, 2007) 41, 42, 49, 103.

102 "demonstrations of the magic art": Blacker, *The Catalpa Bow*, 208.

118 **"With religious beliefs, it can"**: Naoko Kobayashi, "'Nyonin Kinsei' Honto ni Dento nanoka" ("Is 'Women Forbidden' Really a Tradition?"), *Asahi Shimbun*, April 3, 2024, 11.

118 **Japan regularly comes in last:** World Economic Forum, *Global Gender Gap Report 2023*, June 20, 2023, 11, https://www3.weforum.org/docs/WEF_GGGR_2023 .pdf.

119 **"One climbs Mt. Fuji"**: Masaki Sugiyama, "Bi to Shukyuo no Yama ga Unda Fujishinko" ("The Fuji Worship Borne from a Mountain of Beauty and Religion"), *Shukyo Shimbun* (website), accessed September 19, 2024, https://religion-news.net /2023/05/18/sugi799/.

121 **"Should they disobey him," says:** "En no Gyoja to ha" ("About En no Gyoja"), En no Gyoha Reiseki Fudasho Kai, undated, accessed August 12, 2024, http://www.ubasoku.jp /introduction/ennogyoja.htm.

121 **"You will face different trials every time"**: Cameron Allan McKean, "Yamabushi—Yama no gyoja tachi" ("Yamabushi— Yamagata Mountain Ascetics"), *Papersky Japan Stories*, August 12, 2021, accessed August 12, 2024, https://papersky.jp /yamabushi-01/.

CHAPTER 4:
ANGRY GHOSTS: ONRYO

131 **The eighteenth-century religious philosopher Norinaga Motoori:** Norinaga Motoori, *Motoori Norinaga Zenshu* (*The Complete Works of Motoori Norinaga*) (Tokyo: Chikuma Shobô, 1968), vol. 9, 126.

132 **"It was I who wrought the plague"**: *Kojiki* (Kodansha Gakujutsu Bunko, 1980), vol. 2, 86.

134 **"Heaven has granted me a great"**: Giuliana Stramigioli, "Preliminary Notes on Masakadoki and the Taira no Masakado Story," *Monumenta Nipponica* 28, no. 3 (Autumn 1973): 286, accessed June 11, 2024, https://www.jstor.org /stable/2383784.

134 **"Mounted on chargers like dragons":** Stramigioli, "Preliminary Notes," 286.

135 **"Since creation the court has seen":** Karl Friday, *The First Samurai: The Life and Legend of the Warrior Rebel Taira Masakado* (New Jersey: Wiley and Sons, 2008), 9.

138 "SPIRIT OF MASAKADO! WE APOLOGIZE!": *Tokyo Asahi Shimbun*, Evening Edition, March 27, 1928, 2.

147 **A thousand citizens, many dressed in:** Judith N. Rabinovitch, ed., "Shomonki: The Story of Masakado's Rebellion," *Monumenta Nipponica* 58, no. 4 (1986): 3.

CHAPTER 5:
BELIEF WITHOUT BELIEF: HANSHIN-HANGI

155 **Almost 70 percent of Japanese claim:** Hakuhodo Institute of Life and Living, *Shinjiru mono ha nan desu ka? No. 1390: Uranai/omikuji wo shinjinai (What do people believe in? No. 1390: I don't believe in uranai or omikuji)*, accessed June 11, 2024, https://seikatsusoken.jp/teiten/answer/1391.html.

155 **According to surveys, more than half:** Net Research Dimsdrive, *Nenmatsunenshi no sugoshikata ni kan suru ankeeto 2011 (A Survey of How People Spend Year's End and New Year's, 2011)*, accessed June 11, 2024, https://www.dims.ne.jp /timelyresearch/2011/110302/.

155 **"God does play dice with the universe":** Stephen Hawking, "God Does Play Dice" (academic lecture, 1999), accessed June 11, 2024, https://www.hawking.org.uk/in-words/lectures /does-god-play-dice.

165 **At its peak, the magazine's circulation:** Fumito Sakai, *Mai Basudee Soukango ga 1979nen 4gatsu 8ka ni hanbai sareta! (The Inaugural Issue of My Birthday Was Sold on April 8, 1979!)*, accessed August 10, 2024, https://mycale366.jp /post/788.

171 **"In times of old in Japan, worries":** Hiroshi Aramata and Kazuhiko Komatsu, *Sekai wo Yomitoku Uranai to Majinai* ("Deciphering the World Through Fortunes and Spells").

Bessatsu Taiyo: Uranai to Majinai (Fortunes and Spells), Spring 1991, 4–10.

173 **Of the 776 temples and shrines:** "TANTAN no Zatsugaku to Tetsugaku no Koheya" ("TANTAN's Random Philosophy Room"), accessed September 19, 2024, https://information -station.xyz/135.html.

173 **"Uranai can also be seen as":** Aramata et al., *Uranai to Majinai*, 10.

177 **"What am I doing?** *he thought"*: Eiji Yoshikawa, *Musashi: An Epic Novel of the Samurai Era,* trans. Charles S. Terry (Harper & Row/Kodansha International, 1981), 523.

178 **"The Way of the Lone One":** Teruo Machida, "The Last Words of Miyamoto Musashi: An Attempt to Translate His Dokkodo," *Bulletin of the Nippon Sport Science University* 41, no. 2 (2012): 199–211.

CHAPTER 6:
CURATING YOUR RITUALS: FUNERAL BUDDHISM

185 **"The dead don't disappear":** Hideo Kobayashi, *Motoori Norinaga* (Tokyo: Shinchosha Publishing, 1992), 247.

185 **"Architecture, painting, sculpture":** Lafcadio Hearn, *Japan: An Attempt at Interpretation* (New York: Macmillan Company, 1905), 208.

187 **There are 156 schools and sects:** Mariko Kobayashi, ed., *Shyukyo Nenkan (Religious Yearbook)* (Tokyo: Agency of Cultural Affairs, 2023), 8, accessed August 12, 2024, https://www.bunka.go.jp/tokei_hakusho_shuppan/hakusho _nenjihokokusho/shukyo_nenkan/pdf/r05nenkan.pdf.

188 **"a textbook example of religion":** Ryosuke Okamoto, *Shukyo to Nihonjin* (Tokyo: Chuko Shinsho, 2021), 78.

188 **"the formalities of Buddhist memorial":** Okamoto, *Shukyo to Nihonjin*, 76.

189 **Weddings are a huge industry:** "Sales value of the bridal and wedding related market in Japan from 2014 to 2023 with a

forecast for 2024," Statista, April 24, accessed August 12, 2024, https://www.statista.com/statistics/702786/japan-bridal-and-wedding-market-size.

190 **Funerals are a big business:** David McElhinney, "Why Are Japanese Funerals So Expensive?," *Tokyo Weekender*, November 2, 2022, accessed August 10, 2024, https://www.tokyoweekender.com/japan-life/news-and-opinion/japanese-funerals-expensive.

190 **According to one survey, as recently as 2014:** AiNet Group AiNet Hall (website), "Ise Shuhen de no Gososhiki ha Doiu Keishiki ga Ooi no ka?" ("What Kinds of Funerals Are Most Common in the Ise Area?"), May 18, 2020, accessed August 12, 2024, https://isematsusaka-osoushiki.jp/column/detail.html?id=2367.

195 **In February of 2024, a man posted:** User @kj94444018, posted February 22, 2024, accessed February 22, 2024, available at https://twitter.com/kj94444018/status/1760622299114512821?s=58.

198 **Not even my Shinto Cultural Examinations:** Association of Shinto Shrines, *Jinjya no Iroha* (*"All about Jinja"*) (Tokyo: Fusosha Publishing, 2012), 53.

200 **The pioneering folklorist Kunio Yanagita:** This and subsequent quotes on this page are taken from Kunio Yanagita, *Furusato Nana-jyu Nen* (*Seventy Years in My Hometown*), Aozora Bunko website, accessed August 12, 2024, https://www.aozora.gr.jp/cards/001566/files/55742_65234.html.

201 **In a survey from 2007:** Hiromi Shimada, *Soshiki wa Iranai* (*Who Needs Funerals?*) (Tokyo: Gentosha Literary Publication, 2010), 18.

202 **When the husband of a celebrity chef:** Remi Hirano, "Wada san Sogi Sanretsu-sha mo jiipan sugata" ("Mr. Wada's Funeral, Everyone Was in Jeans," *Asahi Shimbun*, April 22, 2021, 3.

207 **"There is no sadness greater":** Kobayashi, *Motoori Norinaga*, 235.

CHAPTER 7:
LOVE WILL TRAVEL: KUYO

216 **"A little Japanese girl does not break her doll":** Lafcadio Hearn, trans., *Japanese Fairy Tale Series No. 25: Chin Chin Kobakama* (Tokyo: T. Hasegawa, 1903).

219 **I've seen *Kuyo* rendered:** George Thomas Bettany, *Primitive Religions: Being an Introduction to the Study of Religions, with an Account of the Religious Beliefs of Uncivilised Peoples, Confucianism, Taoism (China), and Shintoism (Japan)* (England: Ward, Lock & Co., 1891).

223 **Would *The Guardian* have described her:** Anakana Schofield, "What We Gain from Keeping Books—and Why It Doesn't Need to Be 'Joy,'" *The Guardian*, January 7, 2019, accessed August 9, 2024, https://www.theguardian.com/books/2019 /jan/07/what-we-gain-from-keeping-books-and-why-it-doesnt -need-to-be-joy-marie-kondo.

223 ***The New Yorker* have called her:** Troy Patterson, "'Tidying Up with Marie Kondo,' Reviewed: The Organizational Consultant as Freelance Exorcist," *New Yorker*, January 3, 2019, accessed August 9, 2024, https://www.newyorker.com/culture/on -television/tidying-up-with-marie-kondo-reviewed-the -organizational-consultant-as-freelance-exorcist.

223 **around 180,000 groups:** *e-Stat: Seifu Tokei no Sogo Madoguchi (e-Stat: Government Statistics Portal)*, accessed August 9, 2024, https://www.e-stat.go.jp/dbview?sid=0003280702.

223 **In an accompanying report, the agency:** Hiroyuki Mantani, ed., *Shukyo Kanren Tokei ni Kan Suru Shiryoushu (Materials Regarding Religious-Related Statistics)* (Tokyo: Agency for Cultural Affairs, Government of Japan, 2014), 3, accessed August 12, 2024, https://www.bunka.go.jp/tokei_hakusho _shuppan/tokeichosa/shumu_kanrentokei/pdf/h26_chosa .pdf.

224 **our "hodgepodge" spirituality:** Keiji Ueshima, *Kumano Kami to Hotoke (Kumano: Kami and Hotoke)* (Tokyo: Hara Shobo, 2009), 64.

224 **Scholars of the time grappled:** Orion Klautau, "Shukyo Gainen to Nihon" ("Japan and the Concept of Religion"), 246, Graduate School of International Cultural Studies, Tohoku University (website), accessed August 12, 2024, http://web.tohoku.ac.jp/modern-japan/wp-content/uploads/Klautau_Shukyo-Gainen-to-Nihon_2014.pdf.

224 **In books and lectures, critics argued:** Jason Ānanda Josephson, "When Buddhism Became a 'Religion': Religion and Superstition in the Writings of Inoue Enryo," *Japanese Journal of Religious Studies* 33, no. 1: 143–68.

225 **In a 2024 survey, 83 percent of Japanese:** Jonathan Evans et al., *Report, June 17, 2024, Religion and Spirituality in East Asian Societies*, "1. Religious landscape and change," Pew Research Center, accessed August 9, 2024, https://www.pewresearch.org/religion/2024/06/17/religious-landscape-and-change-in-east-asia.

229 **Nearly 10 percent of the over seven hundred universities:** Nobuyuki Kaga, "Kirisuto-kyo Shugi Daigaku (Misshon Sukuuru) Shokai (1) Henshu-bu (Introduction to Christian Universities (Mission Schools) (1) Editorial Department," *Christian Press*, April 17, 2018, accessed August 10, 2024, available at https://christianpress.jp/キリスト教主義大学 (ミッションスクール) 紹介.

CHAPTER 8:
RADICALLY INCLUSIVE: KUMANO

247 **"This route is very rough and difficult":** Tanabe City Kumano Tourist Bureau, eds., "Ogumotori-goe (Koguchi to Nachisan)," undated, accessed August 10, 2024, http://www2.tb-kumano.jp/en/kumano-kodo/pdf/Ogumotori-goe-north-to-south-route-guide.pdf.

247 **The Emperor Go-Shirakawa, who made:** Ryoko Kuraishi, "Bike Packing Weekend: In Pursuit of Spectacular Streams and Odd-Shaped Rocks in the 'Land of Water,'" *Papersky Japan Stories*, July 25, 2022, accessed August 12, 2024,

https://papersky.jp/en/bike-packing-weekend
-wakayama.

250 **It eventually resulted in the outright destruction:** Jørn
Borup, *Japanese Rinzai Zen Buddhism: Myoshinji, a Living
Religion* (Boston: Brill, 2008), 21.

251 **Instead, they forced the yamabushi:** Keiji Ueshima, *Kumano
Kami to Hotoke (Kumano: Kami and Hotoke)* (Tokyo: Hara
Shobo, 2009), 59.

253 **At the time, there was something:** Yorio Fujimoto, *Jinja to
Kamisama ga Yoku Wakaru Hon (The Book for Understanding Jinja
and Kami)* (Tokyo: Shuwa System, 2014), 58.

253 **In that great Meiji rush to modernization:** Manabu Toya,
Jinja to Ekorojii 2 (Jinja and Ecology 2), Nippon.com, November
14, 2016, accessed August 9, 2024, https://www.nippon.com
/ja/views/b05214.

253 **A deluge of water and debris:** Nara Prefecture Land
Management Department, ed., "Kako ni Okotta Nara-ken no
Dosha Saigai" ("Landslide Disasters in Nara Prefecture's
Past"), accessed August 9, 2024, https://www3.pref.nara.jp
/doshasaigai/sabokyouikucontents/manabu_nara.

263 **The mass media repeatedly framed:** Michael Holtz, "In
'Non-Religious' Japan, the Shrine Can Still Exert a Pull,"
Christian Science Monitor (website), September 9, 2015,
accessed September 19, 2024, https://www.csmonitor.com
/World/Asia-Pacific/2015/0906/In-non-religious-Japan-the
-shrine-can-still-exert-a-pull; "Is Religion in Japan in
Irreversible Decline?" *Japan Today* (website), June 12, 2023,
accessed September 19, 2024, https://japantoday.com/
category/features/kuchikomi/is-religion-in-japan-in
-irreversible-decline; Max Fisher and Caitlin Dewey, "A
Surprising Map of Where the World's Atheists Live,"
Washington Post, May 23, 2013.

266 **"When foreigners see Japanese":** Toshinori Tanaka, "Osaka
International Religious Fellowship Anniversary Meeting 2005:
International Symposium 'Water, Forest, Life,'" *Relnet.com*,

accessed August 12, 2024, available at http://www.relnet.co
.jp/kokusyu/brief/kkouen24.htm.

267 **"They took the flood as a sign"**: Ueshima, *Kumano Kami to Hotoke,* 76.

CHAPTER 9:
PRAYER AND PLAY: ASOBI

280 **"We do not have ideology"**: Joseph Campbell, *The Masks of God*, vol. 1, *Oriental Mythology* (New York: Viking Penguin, 1962), 476.

286 **"on either side of the principal temple gate"**: Francis Hall, *Japan through American Eyes: The Journal of Francis Hall, Kanagawa and Yokohama, 1859–1866* (Princeton University Press, 1992), 338.

288 **Up to 30 percent of children perished**: "Nana sai made kami no uchi" ("In the Hands of the Kami Until Age Seven"), Kenji Morita, *Yahoo! Japan News* (website), June 6, 2017, accessed September 19, 2024, https://news.yahoo.co.jp/articles /3e64f99d8925688ffdcf89acdb63b02378798f10.

295 **"It had an eight-forked head"**: Yasumaro no O, *Nihongi: Chronicles of Japan from the Earliest Times to A.D. 697*, vol. 1, trans. William George Aston (London: Kegan Paul, Trench, Trubrer & Co., 1896), 53.

302 **But Ippen developed a distinctive style**: Dennis Hirota, *No Abode: The Record of Ippen* (University of Hawaii Press, 1997), xxxix.

304 **As recently as the 1970s, there were around**: Hidenori Ukai, "Saigo no Itako wo Tazune: Naki Haha to Hanasu" ("Visiting the Last Itako: A Talk with My Departed Mother"), *Nikkei Business*, March 12, 2018, accessed August 10, 2024, https:// business.nikkei.com/atcl/report/16/030500208/030500004.

About the Author

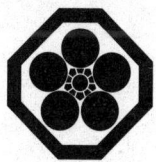

Hiroko Yoda is a certified Shinto cultural historian, a former Tokyo editor for CNNgo, and a field producer for National Geographic TV. Raised in Japan, she earned her master's degree in International Peace and Conflict Resolution from American University in Washington, DC, then embarked on a career of building bridges between East and West. In 2003, she launched the successful pop-culture localization company AltJapan. Her writings have appeared in outlets including CNN, *The New Yorker*, *Wired*, and *T: The New York Times Style Magazine*; and she speaks widely on shows including PBS's *Monstrum* and *99% Invisible*. She is also the coauthor of numerous illustrated books about Japanese folklore, including *Yokai Attack!* and its sequels. She lives in Tokyo.

hirokoyoda.com